# BIOETHICS MEDIATION

*A Guide to Shaping Shared Solutions*

# BIOETHICS MEDIATION

## *A Guide to Shaping Shared Solutions*

Nancy Neveloff Dubler

*and*

Carol B. Liebman

United Hospital Fund of New York

ISBN: 1-881277-704

**Library of Congress Cataloging-in-Publication Data**

Dubler, Nancy N.
   Bioethics mediation : a guide to shaping shared solutions / Nancy Neveloff Dubler and Carol B. Liebman.
      p. ; cm.
Includes bibliographical references and index.
   ISBN 1-881277-70-4
  1. Medical care—Decision making. 2. Mediation. 3. Medical ethics.
   [DNLM: 1. Bioethical Issues. 2. Negotiating—methods. WB 60 D814b 2004]
I. Liebman, Carol B. II. Title. R723.5.D83 2004 174.2—dc22

For information, write, Publications Program, United Hospital Fund of New York, 350 Fifth Avenue, 23rd Floor, New York, NY 10118-2399.

*To our grandchildren*

# Contents

# Foreword

As THE AMERICAN health care system grows more complex, the potential for conflict increases dramatically. Disagreements among health care professionals, patients, and payers are almost inevitable given the growing number of complex choices, compounded by a lack of effective communication between health care professionals and patients and their families, particularly when it comes to grim prognoses and death.

We have never had good ways to deal with conflict in medical settings. And so we were very excited when Nancy Neveloff Dubler approached us with her vision of a new way to approach these conflicts. In the 1980s Ms. Dubler had developed one of the nation's first bioethics consultation services at Montefiore Medical Center in the Bronx. By the early 1990s, she realized that most cases referred to the service were not bioethics dilemmas but conflicts, and that most often the conflict, rather than the bioethical issue, was the key to resolving the case. This insight led Ms. Dubler to another: that mediation and its associated set of dispute resolution skills could be as helpful in the hospital setting as it has proved in resolving complex labor disputes, child custody cases, and even international conflicts.

With grant support from the United Hospital Fund, Ms. Dubler went about figuring out how to apply the mediation model to the medical setting. She enlisted the assistance of expert mediators from around the country for intensive training. The lessons of that early effort were described in *Mediating Bioethical Disputes,* written by Ms. Dubler and Leonard Marcus and published by the United Hospital Fund in 1993.

The current book is enriched by ten years of experience, and the contributions of Carol B. Liebman, a professor of law at Columbia University and herself an expert mediator in diverse settings. Together Ms. Dubler and Ms. Liebman do a masterful job of laying out the theory, background, and practical application of this approach. They make the case for the use of mediation in the health care setting, explain how bioethics mediation differs from traditional mediation, provide a step-by-step approach to the process, and, in rich and nuanced commentary, provide annotated transcripts of mediation sessions.

In keeping with its mission of advancing patient- and family-centered care, the United Hospital Fund has been an enthusiastic supporter of the work of Ms. Dubler and her colleagues in the Division of Bioethics at Montefiore for more than 15 years. In addition to the two publications on bioethics, we published *The Tuberculosis Revival: Individual Rights and Societal Obligations in a Time of AIDS,* by Ms. Dubler, Ronald Bayer, and Sheldon Landesman (1992), which created the conceptual framework for national discussions of this issue. We provided grant support for Montefiore's effort to establish New York City's first post-graduate training program in medical ethics and values for health care professionals and educators. This program, the Certificate Program in Bioethics and Medical Humanities, continues to be a major source of training for health care professionals in New York City and the region. And in 2002 we published *Ethics for Health Care Organizations: Theory, Case Studies, and Tools,* by Jeffrey Blustein, Linda Farber Post, and Ms. Dubler, which describes Montefiore's pioneering effort to establish an institutional code of ethics and outlines how to translate an institution's commitment to a core set of principles into agreed-upon policies and procedures.

We are particularly pleased to have been able to support the current publication, which advances our work to improve the quality of care and to support health care professionals in their efforts to provide the best possible care. It also reinforces important themes that have arisen in our work on palliative care and the role of family caregivers.

From its founding 125 years ago the United Hospital Fund has been shaping positive change in health care. Through its research and analytic work and its programmatic support for projects like Montefiore's, it seeks to shape a health care system that is committed to the highest standards of care and excellence for all New Yorkers.

JAMES R. TALLON, JR.
President

# *Preface*

THIS BOOK IS DESIGNED to help bioethics committees and consultants move from retrospective to prospective consultation. To this end, it provides a conceptual framework with which to analyze cases and introduces the specific tools needed to conduct mediative bioethics interventions. A substantial literature on bioethics consultation has been generated over the past two decades. But whereas different approaches have been identified and discussed, nothing prescriptive has been presented that would help those training for consultation to acquire the interpersonal and process skills that are assumed to be part of the Core Competencies for Health Care Ethics Consultation (American Society for Bioethics and Humanities 1998). We are suggesting, in this book, that although there might be other ways to acquire these skills, by far the most effective and efficient way is to study the body of knowledge, skills, and techniques represented by the field of mediation.

This book also introduces mediators to a little-known use of the mediation process, showing how the process is changed to meet the needs of health care institutions. While the focus here is on the use of mediation to resolve bioethics disputes, we hope both health care providers and mediators will be encouraged to think about other ways in which mediation can be used to facilitate communication and problem solving in health care.

## The Bioethics Consultation Service at Montefiore Medical Center

The Montefiore Bioethics Consultation Service was established in 1978 in response to the growing awareness among medical care providers that legal rights, ethical principles, and moral reasoning are increasingly part of the practice of medicine. The service began with a mandate and a convention. The mandate was to participate in the decision-making process concerning patient care; the convention was to avoid dominating that process. From the outset, the service was intended not to supplant the medical team's input but to foster clearer analysis by applying the reasoning of judicial opinions and ethics scholars to the dilemmas presented in clinical medical practice. In the first years, case interventions were tentative and consisted largely of retrospective analysis in the bioethics committee or with the departments or departmental divisions that had been involved with the case.

Soon, the consult team began to realize that the service provided more than ethical scholarship and legal reasoning. It provided something new and valuable: neutral turf, where clinicians could come together to discuss the patient's medical situation, the likely prognoses, the construction of the family, the relationship of the staff to the patient and the family, and the emotional dynamics of those relationships. Attending physicians, house staff, fellows, residents, students, nurses, social workers, and consultants all sat together and talked about the history, probable future, and past successes and failures of the medical plan. In the course of these conversations, some of the bases for and origins of the dilemmas of care soon emerged. Many times, the tensions between patients, family members, and the medical staff reflected the simple fact that various members of the care team who perceived the medical issues differently had communicated these disparate views to the patient and family and had not discussed them sufficiently within the care team. The result, not surprisingly, was that different family members had adopted different views of the medical facts and the likely prognosis. The inevitable ensuing clashes between and among the family and between and among the care providers regarding how to manage the life, or the death, of the patient were often labeled as bioethics problems and the consulting service was called.

On occasion, the mere fact of bringing all of the far-flung members of the care team together, where they could hear each other and argue their unique perspectives, resulted in an agreement on the likely course of the illness that could then be communicated to the patient or family. Once the conflicting professional messages disappeared, the conflicting family dictates often dissolved as well.

This repeated pattern of resolution led to the theory that this experience might provide a basis for a more self-conscious bioethics intervention process. Specifically, a decade of observation had arrived at a theory: bioethics disputes are essentially conflicts, and the underlying issues of patient and family rights can best be clarified and addressed by approaching the turbulence and discord with the skills of dispute mediators. With this in mind, we enlisted the help of our colleagues from Boston to put this theory into practice.

We asked Dr. Leonard Marcus, Director of the Program for Health Care Negotiation and Conflict Resolution at the Harvard School of Public Health, and David Matz, a member of The Mediation Group and Director of the Graduate Program in Dispute Resolution at the University of Massachusetts at Boston, to train the bioethics consultation team, the risk managers (who often dealt with facets of the same disputes), and colleagues from the American Bar Association Commission on the Legal Problems of the Elderly (who were increasingly interested in dispute resolution) in techniques of mediation. The project was funded by the United Hospital Fund, the publisher of this book and an ongoing supporter of our efforts in this realm.

The collaboration between bioethics and mediation professionals was not always easy. We began the first day's training by focusing on a common scenario: the capable patient who wants to refuse life-sustaining care but whose wife wants him to accept treatment and live. Legally and ethically, a patient who is capable of making decisions has the right to refuse care even if the result of that refusal is death—so, a bioethicist might ask, what is left for negotiation or mediation? But as the mediation professionals pointed out, that assumption reflects the naïve notion that matters of legal rights and ethical interests play out in clarity and calm. In reality, the fact that a patient has a right to decide may not dictate that the patient has the emotional strength to insist on that right in the face of a family member's[1] concerned opposition. And in mediation, our mentors noted, the process is part of the product. The goal of this first scenario was to arrive at the conclusion that the patient had the right to decide. A secondary goal was to help his wife and the care team understand and support his decision.

After undergoing mediation training, we no longer had any doubt that mediation offers an appealing enhancement to bioethics consultation. It acknowledges the primacy of rights and the complexity of interests in medical care decision making. It recognizes the differentials in power and authority that pervade the medical setting. Most important, it has established skills and a body of knowledge that can be brought to bear on difficult, sometimes seemingly intractable, disputes.

When bioethics mediation programs were getting started, many bioethicists were reluctant to use the term "mediation" because it characterizes the event as a "conflict" when it has not been so designated by the parties. When staff disagree about the course to follow, they generally perceive their disagreement as the search for the "best outcome" or the care plan that is in the "best interest" of the patient. Many physicians and nurses and also many family members would be shocked by the suggestion that their disagreements have risen to the level of conflict, although in many cases that would be a correct portrayal.

---

1. When we say "family members" we mean to include not just the patient's biological family but also all beloved others (Levine and Zuckerman 1999).

In some cases, however, identifying the conflict as a conflict actually helps to clear the air by clarifying the issues, defusing some of the political and hierarchical power-trips that sometimes surround conflict, and empowering the less dominant and influential of the staff to speak up and voice their concerns. Moreover, calling the session a mediation may make it easier for the mediator to "import" experts without bruising any egos, because that designation may be cited as the basis for the request for additional or new information.

There may be an additional argument for calling the session a mediation. Many states have passed legislation protecting the confidentiality of mediation communications. Some statutes make mediation communications inadmissible in litigation and administrative proceedings, while others create a privilege for mediation communication. Especially in highly contentious mediations, knowing that what is said in the mediation cannot "be used against" any of the participants in future proceedings should the mediation not help the parties reach agreement can be critical to open, candid discussion.[2]

Thus, we developed the process of mediating bioethics disputes (Dubler and Marcus 1994), and mediation has been an integral part of the Montefiore Bioethics Consultation Service ever since. Our services are available to physicians, nurses, social workers, house staff, medical students, family members, and patients who have been troubled by the decision-making process, the values reflected, or the interests imperiled in a case. Any member of the medical team can request a consultation, as long as the attending physician, who is legally responsible for the care of the patient, is alerted immediately and offered a key place in the discussion.

In dealing with approximately one hundred consultations a year for many years, we have found that there is always a "bioethics hook" on which to hang the initial request for a consultation. However, when the situation is investigated, it is clear that most cases referred to the Bioethics Consultation Service are not really bioethics dilemmas but conflicts that have been defined in bioethics language—and most often the conflict rather than the bioethical issue becomes the key to the case. Thus, bioethics consultation is largely, although not entirely, a matter of conflict resolution. And, while bioethics consultants certainly need to be experts in the ethical, legal, and medical issues, they also should have a good grasp of a governing process and a strong set of dispute resolution skills.

---

2. Nonetheless, it must be made clear to all participants that key aspects of the discussion might need to be reflected in a chart note that would be discoverable in any future legal actions, since it is an open, accessible part of the hospital care plan; a promise of any protection might be misleading.

Each case presented in the following chapters has a bioethics issue that defined the presenting problem: the family is demanding care that is not in the best interest of the patient; the family, in derogation of a living will, wants "everything done" for the patient; the patient is refusing care and is not capable of making that decision; or the physician is insisting on care that the family claims the patient would refuse if the patient were capable. These are "bioethics hooks," but in and of themselves they say nothing ethically critical about the case or its likely outcome. What they do signal, and very clearly, is that conflict surrounds the case.

This book is the result of the extensive collaboration and mutually supportive learning that have engaged the co-authors in the past seven years. The catalyst for this shared experience was the spring-semester retreat of the Certificate Program in Bioethics and Medical Humanities (a joint program of Montefiore Medical Center and the New York University Division of Nursing). The spring training in mediation had been held twice, and the first book on mediating bioethical disputes had been published (Dubler and Marcus 1994), when Nancy Dubler and Carol Liebman linked efforts. What Dubler brought to the project was the notion that these dilemmas could be approached more systematically; what Liebman brought was the intellectual framework for a systematic assessment and intervention. What we could do together was, over the years, test the theory in the crucible of hospital reality—defining, honing, and recalibrating the theory and practice as experience dictated.

The work of the Montefiore Medical Center Bioethics Consultation Service has given us ample opportunity to test this theory. The business of consultation is gratifying and humbling. We have not presented the easy victories; those are not very interesting. We have agreed, and our consult notes demonstrate, that getting the parties together, airing views, clarifying and sharing different perspectives normally results in a care plan with which all of the parties can be comfortable. The cases presented here show how hard the process can be and how often it can fail despite what we would suggest is a principled approach to the issues and the process.

## The Structure of This Book

*Part I. A Framework for Understanding Bioethics Mediation* (Chapters 1–2) demonstrates the value of mediation as a tool for addressing the complex conflicts encountered in the medical context. It distills and analyzes the experience of an active bioethics consultation service in a large urban teaching hospital over the past decade—encounters, learning, successes, and failures—using a combination of cases and scholarly discussions. (In every description of a case, the names have been changed and the medical histories altered to protect the privacy of the patients, families, and care providers.) These chapters provide essential background for parties preparing to engage in bioethics mediation.

*Part II. A Practical Guide to Bioethics Mediation* (Chapters 3–5) provides a detailed guide to preparing for and conducting effective bioethics mediations. The methods and steps presented combine the lessons of actual consultations in the medical setting with the literature of mediation and the training of professional mediators.

*Part III. Case Analyses* (Chapters 6–8) presents examples of the complex and humbling cases encountered by bioethics consultants. These cases underscore the need for a dynamic approach to bioethics consultation; principles are the starting points for consultation, but in and of themselves, they are incapable of resolving the conflicts that surround care. Mediation theory and practice can offer the necessary intellectual grounding and technical skills.

*Part IV. Role Plays: Practicing Mediation Skills* (Chapters 9–12) provides fresh material for people working in institutional settings to develop and practice their skills in bioethics mediation by role playing as members of bioethics mediation teams. Each chapter outlines a case and provides individual instructions for participants. Each case presents a fresh configuration of the needs and wants of the patient or family members in the context of medical care options. And each case is different—but understanding and trying out the principles and practices suggested in this book will help professionals in real-life bioethics conflicts to maneuver most effectively toward a solution.

*Part V. Annotated Transcripts of Bioethics Mediation Role Plays* (Chapters 13–14) provides annotated transcripts of actual role-playing sessions that used the material presented in Chapters 10 and 11. The sessions were recorded during one of the spring-semester retreats on mediating bioethics disputes that takes place annually in the Certificate Program in Bioethics and Medical Humanities.

# Acknowledgments

ALTHOUGH THIS BOOK is primarily the collaboration of Nancy Dubler and Carol Liebman, it has been enriched by the experience and wisdom of colleagues, scholars, and practitioners. A few need special thanks. Barbara Swartz, Bruce K. Gould Distinguished Professor at Touro Law School, a scholar of health law, and an expert mediator, was on sabbatical at the Montefiore Medical Center Division of Bioethics in 1999. She provided mentorship and inspiration, read drafts of the book, and participated in a set of mediations. Her comments on those mediations provided the basis for an instant critique of the process and product. Her notes and comments on some of the cases are integrated into Chapters 6, 7, and 8.

Leslie Bailey arrived at our doorstep as a summer intern after her first year at New York University Law School. Her first project was to help us think through the task of weaving together the writing, thinking, assumptions, and styles of two academics in very different settings, with vastly different experience. Luckily for us, Leslie was gifted in the way she attacked her tasks and organized her material. She was also amiable and dogged: without her skill and good humor this book might never have emerged.

In that same year Marc Fleischer was a fellow in the division. He and Chris Stern Hyman participated with Professor Swartz in a working group on the topic "What Counts as Evidence in Bioethics Mediation?" The fruits of this discussion are most visible in Chapter 3. An earlier form of the chapter, entitled, "What Counts as 'Evidence' in Mediating Bioethical Disputes?" was presented at the conference, "What Is *Your* Evidence? Defending Arguments in a Pluralistic World," the Fourth Annual Seminar, Centre for Values, Ethics, and the Law in Medicine at the University of Sydney, Australia, August 2000. Also in Australia, Professors Miles Little and Bernadette Tobin provided critical and constructive suggestions.

Jeffrey Blustein and Linda Farber Post, at the Montefiore Division of Bioethics, have been unfailingly generous with their time and energy and have read and commented on multiple drafts of this book. Their experience with the reality of mediating bioethical disputes in the day-to-day work of the Bioethics Consultation

Service provided a depth of wisdom and understanding that infuses the narratives and commentaries. Tia Powell was a critical reader who provided a mid-course correction for the final draft. Margaret Shaw and Ellen Waldman generously spent time reviewing an earlier stage of the book and making thoughtful and wise suggestions.

Many of the issues discussed and the techniques presented had their origins in the first Montefiore Mediation Project in 1992. Two members of the American Bar Association Commission on Law and Aging, Erica Wood and Naomi Karp, participated in that project and have been thoughtful colleagues on mediation issues since that time.

The mentors for that project were Leonard Marcus and David Matz. They were generous with their time and energies. Leonard Marcus and Nancy Dubler wrote the first book on the subject, *Mediating Bioethical Disputes* (Dubler and Marcus 1994). That first project and the subsequent publication were supported by grants from the United Hospital Fund, an early, enthusiastic, and ongoing supporter of the work of Nancy Dubler and the Division of Bioethics.

The model of bioethics mediation presented here benefited greatly from the insights of the teaching team members of the weekend retreat on mediation of the Certificate Program in Bioethics and Medical Humanities, a joint project of the Division of Bioethics and the Division of Nursing at New York University: David Geronemus, Paul Sarkozi, Marc Fleischer, Jean Miller, Chris Stern Hyman, and, especially, Ann Bensinger. The role play scripts in Part IV were developed for that retreat. Mathy Mezey, co-director of the Certificate Program with Nancy Dubler for the past six years, was an invaluable colleague in the process.

Our great thanks to the clinical and administrative staff at Montefiore Medical Center. These nurses, physicians, and social workers are unfailingly open to new ideas and always searching for ways to improve patient care. They have been critically available to new ways of thinking about communication and dispute resolution. Special thanks to Leslie Carrington, assistant to the Division of Bioethics, who keeps track of consultations—and everything else that moves throughout the division—with efficiency and good humor. Thanks also to the Columbia Law School Clinic staff, Brenda Eberhart, Athena Vagelatos, Vanessa Salazar, and Shavonne Norris for their patient and cheerful assistance.

A special category of thanks goes to Phyllis Brooks, our editor at the United Hospital Fund. Her vision, abiding commitment, and extraordinary skills moved the book from fledgling idea to reality.

Finally, we thank our husbands, Walter and Lance, who read drafts, offered advice, and provided copious amounts of wine and chocolate when appropriate or necessary.

# I

# A FRAMEWORK FOR UNDERSTANDING BIOETHICS MEDIATION

*This part explores the notion of mediation and why it seems so appropriate to the issue of bioethics consultation. All professionals who engage in bioethics consultation would agree that process skills and interpersonal skills are necessary for the person directing the consultation (American Society for Bioethics and Humanities 1998, 14). Whereas mediation has been proposed as one perspective for training professionals and conducting a consultation, we would like to suggest that it is the best theoretical framework in which to embed these tasks:*

- *Mediation is a body of knowledge and a set of skills that can be taught.*
- *Skilled mediators are available to provide training and can be linked with bioethics professionals in mutually supportive relationships.*
- *Mediation is more and more interesting, at least to those professionals who see the imposition of administrative directives as an unappealing outcome of conflict over care plans.*
- *Risk-managers and litigation experts increasingly agree that poor communication with the patient and family is hazardous in terms of later possible litigation and that mediation provides a route to structure and guide that communication.*
- *Mediation provides a scholarly literature that can be linked with bioethics consultation and thus enrich the field.*

*In making this argument we deconstructed the discussion into as many of the component parts as we could in an effort to raise all of the issues that might confront the busy and harried bioethics mediator in a contemporary health care setting.*

# 1

## Why Mediation?

### The Isolated Wife Adjusting to Loss: Edward Davidoff's Case

Edward Davidoff, an 82-year-old man, was admitted to the cardiac service with chest pain. Diagnostic tests revealed the need for quadruple bypass surgery to open four occluded vessels. He was a poor candidate for surgery, however, because he had chronic uncontrolled diabetes with moderate-to-severe compromise of his peripheral vascular system. Unfortunately, there were no other choices if he wanted to live, which he did, and surgery was performed.

After the surgery, Mr. Davidoff did not recover and developed various infections, necessitating his return to surgery for the removal of infected muscle and bone. A bioethics consultation was requested after the second surgery, at which time he was ventilator-dependent with an open chest wound that would not heal. Mr. Davidoff's wife was desperate about her husband's condition and determined that he should recover. She was unable to assimilate the nuanced, and not very clear, discussion by the care team, which used euphemisms to indicate that Mr. Davidoff was dying. No one in the cardiac team had been blunt about the prognosis and Mrs. Davidoff used this oblique discourse to reinforce her own unrealistic expectations about her husband's possible recovery. Completely alone and desperately lonely, she had moved her chair out into the hall and sat there waiting to waylay any staff member who came along who had any connection to the care of her husband. She responded to any specific discussion about care options by choosing the most invasive option (why that option had been presented was the first question the bioethics mediator asked the cardiac team), which she equated with the best chance of insuring her husband's survival. She was never told directly that his survival would be unprecedented, and so it is not surprising that she continued to demand that "everything be done." This demand led to the request for a consultation.

The consult was called by the nursing supervisor, who had been spending increasing time with Mrs. Davidoff. In keeping with the usual procedure of the service, the bioethics mediator met first with the care team—the cardiothoracic surgeon, the vascular surgeon, the first- and second-year residents, the surgical fellows, the primary nurse, and the nursing supervisor. They discussed the case and explored the history of Mr. Davidoff's care and the prognosis, concurring that Mr. Davidoff was unlikely to survive the night. No one had yet communicated this prognosis to Mrs. Davidoff. Moreover, Mr. Davidoff had clearly stated to various members of the care team that if the surgery failed, he did "not want to be kept alive on machines."

The team felt that it had an obligation to the oft-expressed wishes of the patient but also to the grieving of the wife. The team members did not think that Mrs. Davidoff could manage to decide to remove her husband from the ventilator, although they felt that removal was probably what Mr. Davidoff would have wanted. Furthermore, they felt that a do not resuscitate (DNR) order was needed to prevent a terrible death if Mr. Davidoff went into cardiac arrest. The open chest wound precluded any effective resuscitation effort.

Before ending the care team discussion, the mediator asked which members of the large team wanted to be part of the discussion with the patient's wife; confronting her with the entire group would be intimidating. It was agreed that the cardiothoracic surgeon, one of the surgical fellows, one of the residents, and the primary nurse would meet with her. The mediator next asked who should lead the discussion. She explained that she was a "stranger" to the patient's wife and would introduce herself and explain her role but that she need not lead the discussion unless that was the wish of the team members. They asked her to lead the discussion.

The primary nurse then invited Mrs. Davidoff to join this smaller team. The mediator introduced herself and explained her role. "Sometimes when members of the care team and members of the family disagree about a plan of care," she said, "I am invited to join the discussion. My role is not to make the decision but rather to explore the various options—first with the care team, and later with the team and the family—to see whether all can reach a consensus about the best care plan for the patient. I am sort of a mediator but I am an employee of the hospital. I have spoken with the care team and they seem to think that your husband is dying."

"You mean like in a year or six months?" Mrs. Davidoff asked.

"No," the mediator answered, "maybe even today. They have not been able to remove the infection, which continues to spread, and they seem to think that there is not much more that they can do. They are also concerned about the fact that your husband told many of them that if he were

in a state where he was on machines and where he was not expected to recover he would want to be permitted to die." She went on to explain the
team's reasons for wanting to remove Mr. Davidoff from the ventilator and
why they recommended a DNR order.

Mrs. Davidoff had no involved family and only a few friends, none of
whom came with her to the hospital. Also, she was Jewish and it was the
time of Rosh Hashanah, the Jewish New Year, when families often get together and when, by religious tradition, decisions about life and death are
logged for the future year. For any person accustomed to this practice, it is
a time when being alone would be particularly poignant. Mrs. Davidoff
therefore requested the support of a rabbi and soon agreed that her husband would not want to live this way and that a supportive care plan was
appropriate.

BIOETHICS CONFLICTS range in difficulty from simple to extremely complex.
This book emphasizes difficult cases, to illustrate the range of issues involved in me-
diating complex disputes. But the majority of bioethics conflicts are similar to Mr.
Davidoff's case and fall at the easier end of the spectrum.

In Mr. Davidoff's case the fragmentation of the care team, the complexity of the
prognosis, the disinclination of medical staff to talk about death, and the unrealistic hopes of his wife combined to produce a conflict about the best plan of care.
Although cases like this one may raise bioethical issues, the skills that are called
into play—helping those most concerned about the patient clarify the medical
facts, explore the options, and develop solutions that reflect the patient's values
and satisfy the family—are most often associated with classical mediation. The distinctive character of clinical bioethics consultation creates its own process, however,
blending ethical principles and mediative skills into something unique. This unique
process is the subject of this book.

## Managing Conflict in the Contemporary Medical Context

Bioethics is about people: the lives and deaths of individual patients in the context
of family, friends, and care providers—and the personalities, history, attitudes, and
feelings, including fears and a sense of guilt, and the commitments of each person
involved (see box, p. 6). In recent years, bioethics disputes have become more common. Both the patients' rights movement and the consumer movement have legit-
imized the place of the family and the patient in deliberations regarding medical
matters. At the same time, awareness of the potential for conflict has grown as a

### What Is Bioethics?

Bioethics is a body of scholarship produced by philosophers, lawyers, medical care providers, and theologians who, in a dialogue over the past few decades, have identified shared values that provide the basis for normative principles and rules. These normative statements have been derived from benchmark ethical theory, largely propounded by John Stuart Mill and Immanuel Kant, that deals with interlocking ideas about morality and human behavior.

Bioethics also involves a set of ethical principles that support the therapeutic relationship and give rise to physician and caregiver obligations. These include patient autonomy (supporting and facilitating the capable patient's exercise of self-determination); beneficence (promoting the patient's best interest and well-being and protecting the patient from harm); nonmaleficence (avoiding doing harm to the patient); and distributive justice (allocating fairly the benefits and burdens related to health care delivery). (See pp. 36–37 for a fuller discussion of these important ethical principles.) Finally, bioethics is about legal rules that have been created by courts and legislative bodies at the federal and state levels. These rules have recognized and responded to the developing practices in medicine.

result of the shifting structure of health care funding and delivery. The growth of managed care and the shift from fee-for-service medicine (with its incentives for overtreatment) to capitated arrangements (with their incentives for undertreatment) have fueled a growing mistrust among patients and their families, who perceive that the integrity of the care provided may be affected by factors external to the best interests of the patient. This shift has also led to increased tension between doctors and nurses, on the one hand, and organizational administrators, on the other, who seek to improve the profitability of the health care institution by increasing the productivity of health care providers and shortening the time patients spend in acute care institutions. As a result of these changes—and of the ever-increasing number of medical choices available—bioethics consultation has taken on a heightened profile, reflected in the developing professionalism of the field, the growth of graduate school programs, the increase in the number and quality of scholarly publications and academic programs that prepare professionals for the tasks of clinical bioethics, and the impact of national organizations (see box, p. 7).

In 1992, the Joint Commission on Accreditation of Healthcare Organizations established a new standard that required all accredited institutions to have the capacity to address ethical issues in medical care and practice. The result of that pro-

### Styles of Bioethics Consultation

Professionals with expertise in biomedical ethics either chair or advise ethics committees, present monthly seminars, participate in psychosocial rounds and conferences, offer grand rounds, and teach in medical, nursing, and allied health professional schools and other academic settings.

The most common mode of bioethics consultation is the "teaching round," which incorporates the bioethics professional into the structure for assessing patients and discussing their care. During these bedside rounds, a bioethicist will focus on the present state of the "medical facts," especially those aspects of the patient's condition that are relevant to his or her capacity to provide ethically and legally valid informed consent. The bioethicist will also inquire about advance directives and will likely ask about the configuration of the family.

When called in as a consultant on a case, a bioethicist will review the medical chart, talk to staff and family, and then either communicate an opinion to the attending physician or write a consult note in the chart. This style is most akin to the tradition of general medical consultation in which the consultant, whether in gastroenterology or infectious disease, applies his or her specific skill and experience to the medical facts of the case. It remains the obligation and responsibility of the attending physician to evaluate the knowledge brought by the consultant and integrate the consultations into the care of the patient.

nouncement was the creation of a new wave of ethics committees, which sought to develop the capacities to engage in case consultation, education, and policy development.

It would be difficult now to find a health care institution of any quality that does not have an ethics committee addressing staff education, policy protocols, and, at the very least, retrospective case consultation or review. In their formative stages, most bioethics committees engaged in retrospective analysis as a way of educating themselves about the conflicts that exist in clinical practice. As they have become more sophisticated, these committees have increasingly become involved in real-time discussions that affect the outcome of patient care decisions under way. In 1998, the American Society for Bioethics and Humanities (1998, 2) developed a set of core competencies for bioethics consultation that detail the qualifications bioethics consultants must possess in order to operate prospectively and intervene in developing cases.

But just how to move forward was a puzzle to many committees and fledgling consultation efforts. Intervening in cases as they evolve, and by intervening perhaps changing the medical plan, brings with it the need for a theory of practice to guide the intervention. Analyzing what has happened in the past has fewer moral consequences than helping to determine what will happen in the future. Should the consultant or small group advise the caregivers? Should they write their opinions in the chart? Should they intervene in the care plan being developed? Should they impose their values and notions of the "right" and the "good" on the caregiving team? And how should the patient's family be involved in these discussions? Consultations often address issues, such as the withdrawal of treatment or the limitation of care, although they may equally well suggest a more aggressive care plan. One cannot and should not be prepared to intervene in this process of decision making without having clear notions of the governing principles and procedural guidelines that will structure and constrain the intervention.

This book is an attempt to answer those questions within a frame that we think is just, fair, and effective. As long as disparate values exist within families and between patients, families, and the health care system, conflicts are inevitable. And if conflicts are inevitable, strategies for managing them are required—both morally and practically. This book proposes that the best process for identifying, understanding, and resolving conflicts in bioethics consultations is a *mediative intervention*. Such a process identifies the parties to the conflict, clarifies the medical facts, helps the patient and, if involved, the family to amplify the values and interests of the patient in the complex and intimidating structure of the medical center, and helps the parties determine whether there is space for a shared resolution.

## Mediation

Mediation has been used since ancient times to resolve disputes. It is a private, voluntary, informal process in which an impartial third person facilitates a negotiation between people in conflict and helps them find solutions that meet their interests and needs. The current alternative dispute resolution movement began in the late 1960s and early 1970s with impetus from two very different sources. In many areas community action groups turned to mediation as a way to draw on local people and local values to resolve conflicts. The focus was on shaping outcomes that met community interests and that provided a higher quality outcome than was likely to result from a formal process. At about the same time courts began to look to mediation as a docket management tool, focusing on the opportunity for a more efficient and more economical resolution of cases, rather than on ways in which mediation could enhance the quality of the resolution. Today mediators are routinely consulted in employment cases, special education cases, and civil cases ranging from the most complex to those in small-claims court. They are called on to help resolve family disputes (divorce, custody and visitation, parent-child, and estate cases), consumer disputes, environmental disputes, and labor-management disputes, as well as disputes within institutions as diverse as junior and senior high schools and the U.S. Postal Service. On the international level mediators have been called on to help restore peace or avoid violent conflict.

The mediator works with the parties, helping them identify their goals and priorities, generate and explore options, and exchange information that may be necessary for formulating a solution. Unlike a judge or arbitrator, the mediator is not interested in acquiring information in order to determine what happened and who is to blame, nor does a mediator decide who is right and who is wrong or impose solutions on the parties.[1] In mediation the historical facts are important only insofar as they give the mediator and the parties an understanding of how each of them experienced the event that brought them to mediation. Another way to conceptualize the difference between mediation and adjudication is to think of mediation as a process that allows the discovery of that version—or interpretation—of reality that can accommodate the coinciding and conflicting interests and needs of the participating parties.

Mediation is based on three core principles: party autonomy, informed decision making, and confidentiality. Mediators are optimists. They believe most people enmeshed in a conflict have the ability, given the proper setting and access to necessary information, to consider options and select resolutions that meet their needs. Confidentiality allows the parties to speak freely, without fear that what they say during the mediation will have repercussions in a subsequent proceeding.[2]

Introducing a mediator into a dispute does not change the fact that the participants are essentially involved in a negotiation process. A large part of the value added by a mediator is in serving as a guide and coach, helping the disputants move from position-based to interest-based negotiation,[3] encouraging them to discover solutions in which value is not left on the table and each realizes as many of his or her goals as possible, focusing the parties on interests, discovering differences in preferences, and helping them generate options.

---

1. The mediator is interested, however, in learning each party's view of what happened in order to have a better understanding of the issues that should be addressed, not to determine whose version of the facts is "true."

2. In the health care context, however, confidentiality is limited. The health care team shares all medically necessary information. See Chapter 2.

3. See Fisher and Ury 1981 for a discussion of the difference between positions and interests.

## Mediation in Health Care Settings

In the hospital setting, where health care providers, faced with intense demands on their time, are called on to explain complex information and deliver bad news to physically and emotionally vulnerable patients and their families and where large numbers of physicians, nurses, and other providers interact with one another and with the patient, it is not surprising that communication breaks down and disputes arise. Mediation is now used in a variety of medical settings to deal with disputes between residents and staff in nursing homes, disputes over Medicare reimbursement, and quality-of-care complaints involving Medicare and Medicaid, and to resolve medical malpractice claims and bioethics disputes, most notably by Montefiore Medical Center in its pioneering program. Bioethics mediation combines the clinical substance and perspective of bioethics consultation with the tools of the mediation process, using the techniques of mediation and dispute resolution in order to:

- identify the parties to the conflict (although disagreements between family and care providers are common, most conflicts have more than two sides);
- understand the stated (presented) and latent interests of the participants;
- level the playing field to minimize disparities of power, knowledge, skill, and experience (to the degree possible) that separate medical professional, patient, and family;
- help the parties define their interests;
- help maximize options for a resolution of the conflict;
- search for common ground or areas of consensus;
- ensure that the consensus can be justified as a "principled resolution," compatible with the principles of bioethics and the legal rights of patients and families;
- help to implement the agreement; and
- conduct follow-up.

Bioethics mediation in the acute care setting can serve many ends. It may, under certain circumstances, enhance the autonomy of the patient, support the shared values of patient and family, or make clear and strengthen the agreed-upon principles of health care provision. Sometimes it results in the implementation of a commonly shared plan. Whatever the end result, the fundamental goal of mediating bioethics disputes is to maximize the likelihood that a principled resolution (see box) will be reached, in a way that is comfortable for all parties.

---

### *Principled Resolution*

A principled resolution is a plan that falls within clearly accepted ethical principles, legal stipulations, and moral rules defined by ethical discourse, legislatures, and courts and that facilitates a clear plan for future intervention.

---

A key component of bioethics mediation is the creation of "neutral turf," made possible by the presence of a person who is not a member of the health care team and who has not participated in the interventions that have gone awry or the discussions that have broken down. Unlike the classical mediator, who is assumed to be totally impartial and is not connected to either party, the bioethics mediator will likely be an employee of the hospital that is the site of the dispute. Nonetheless, the bioethics mediator brings a distinct set of concerns and skills to the meetings with providers, patients, and family and must be impartial to the situation at hand.

One important reason for a bioethics mediation is to "level the playing field" and give patients and families opportunities to be heard. Frequently, in the context of modern medical facilities, the patient's voice is muted, if not lost, and the patient's ability to vindicate his or her interests is overpowered. The power imbalance in a hospital setting comes from many sources: the difference in level of knowledge and expertise between most patients and the treatment team, the highly technical and unfamiliar physical setting, and the imperfectly aligned interests of the patient and the treatment team members.

The physical and emotional stress of serious illness also contributes to an uneven playing field. Patients in hospitals are often very sick; cognition, understanding, and judgment are all affected by illness. Some patients regress when ill and become dependent. Others simply withdraw. Also, families are under moderate to extraordinary stress depending on the health status of the patient and on the trajectory of illness—whether the patient is improving or deteriorating. A family's ability to cope with hard decisions depends on long-established patterns. Families with a tradition of pulling together and supporting each other will do better than families with histories of discord. Dysfunctional families rarely improve under stress.

Families under stress are at a disadvantage in medical settings also because they have a bad collective reputation among health care professionals (Symposium 1999;

esp. Powell 1999). They are regarded as disruptive, hard to manage, and at odds with staff, although there are almost no hard data to support these opinions or prejudices.

Often families feel that no one has really listened to them or taken their wishes and concerns into consideration. They may not believe that they are viewed as an active and integral part of the process by the medical staff. Sometimes the very fact that they are able to express themselves in an environment where they feel their views are respected can be more meaningful than reaching the solution they had first advocated. If families feel they have been heard, they may be more open when listening to the concerns of the medical staff and more willing to work with them to find the most satisfactory treatment options for the patient.

One of the greatest advantages of using the mediation process in bioethics disputes is that the process is flexible. The general structure of mediation can be adapted and altered to fit the needs of the participants. But the starting point is always the same: respect for the patient, the family, and the care providers and an impartial stance regarding what should be the outcome in any particular case.

In bioethics mediation, the process is a key part of the product. Opening up the decision for scrutiny by a larger, medically sophisticated group and for the recognition of interested parties who have relevant information and relevant value considerations is, in and of itself, a step ahead in the ethical process. It is much harder to take any action that skirts ethical norms when many people are alerted to the problem and are watching the outcome. In this sense, bioethics mediation is of value because it permits a problem to be characterized and analyzed by a greater number of trained professionals, thereby collecting experience and facilitating multidisciplinary discussion. This fact also makes it less likely that the bioethics consultant will be co-opted by the more powerful players in the medical center. Bioethics consultation, when effected through the process of mediation, is collaborative and open. The bias of this book is that collaborative processes are, by their very nature, superior to secret, hidden, authoritarian, and private decision making that emerges only as a progress note or a consultant script in the medical chart. The openness inherent in mediation is one of its chief strengths.

## The Limitations of Mediation

Mediation does not always succeed. Indeed, this book describes some real-life cases where it did not (see Chapters 6 and 8). Various characteristics of conflict may combine to make mediation impossible in a particular circumstance. Parties to a mediation must want to reach agreement. Thus, if a physician has strongly held religious beliefs, value preferences, or practice patterns that are rigid and conflict with the values and desires of the patient, the patient might need to capitulate or shift his or her care to a different physician. Implacable opposition to patient or family choice might mean that the bioethics mediator must shift the discussion of the underlying policy issue to a different forum, either an institutional bioethics committee or a properly empowered administrative person or body. In some cases, the patient or family members may not have the emotional strength to take responsibility for facing difficult facts or making hard choices. They may need to have some decisions made for them. When mediation does not result in an agreement, it is useful to remember that the impasse may not be a sign of failure but, most likely, an indicator that another process is better suited to resolving the dispute. Moreover, participation in the process may have given participants the opportunity to exchange information, clarify goals, and explore options that will aid in finding resolution in some other forum.

## Mediation and Consultation Distinguished

Sometimes in bioethics mediation the mediator will need to step out of the role of mediator and into the role of consultant. This role switch is most likely to happen if the process is leading to an ethically unsupportable outcome. For example, the mediator may need to stop the discussion to explain and support certain norms of decisions and of care and to suggest a principled analysis leading to a solution.[4] Bioethics mediators always wear two hats. They are seekers for the resolution of the conflict (mediator) and, at the same time, transmitters of an accepted body of knowledge that may constrain a solution in any individual case (consultant) (see the box on the next page). Indeed, it is precisely because of the distinctive quality of bioethics disputes and the demands of the clinical setting that the process is better characterized as a clinical intervention than as an administrative procedure.

---

4. In the mediation world the term "med-arb" (mediation-arbitration) is used to describe a process in which the mediator changes roles and becomes the decision maker when the parties are unable to reach agreement. This process is controversial (and disfavored by the authors) because the knowledge that the neutral mediator may ultimately pass judgment on what he or she has heard is likely to affect what the participants say to the mediator and how they say it and also the type of information the mediator elicits and to which he or she attends.

---

### *Bioethics Mediation and Bioethics Consultation*

Bioethics mediation is different from bioethics consultation. *Bioethics consultation* refers to a directed substantive process. The consultant listens to the parties and helps move them toward a principled resolution of the dispute by explaining ethical principles and legal rules, applying them to the facts, and presenting the social consensus on the permissibility of different practices. *Bioethics mediation* refers to the use of classical mediation techniques to identify, understand, and resolve conflicts. Bioethics mediation and bioethics consultation may both be employed in a particular case at different points in the process. Mediation is more inclusive and empowering, and consultation is more authoritarian and hierarchical; either or both may be required in any complex case, even within a single meeting.

---

## The Case for Mediation

In the medical world there is some controversy about the appropriateness of mediation as a model for bioethics consultation. Is bioethics mediation truly mediation? Or is it just the imposition of the staff's will, through the supposedly neutral mediator, on patients and families? It could be charged that the bioethics mediator simply enforces the dominant norm and does not act as a neutral participant in an even-handed process.

This book, however, presents an alternative, more sympathetic interpretation. The reality is that bioethics consultation is generally called for only in difficult cases. In cases where the family, patient, and care providers agree on the diagnosis, prognosis, and care plan going forward, there is no real need for a bioethics consultation.

In difficult cases, the real question is, which is the "least bad" process for drawing out and resolving the issues? The bioethics consultant could decide what is the "right" ethically and legally based solution in the case; the attending physician could decide what, in his or her professional opinion, is the best medical plan; or an administrator, usually a risk manager, could determine what outcome would put the institution in the least dangerous position in terms of possible future liability. But the bioethics mediator, in contrast, would ensure that the options are based on respect for persons, respect for interests and rights of patients and families, and regard for differences. To remove the discussion from the realm of family interaction and merely let the hospital make the decisions would be an authoritarian resolution. Such resolutions, happily, are rare. To see how a bioethics mediation can frame the discussion, allow the family to have their values, hopes, and fears heard, and constrain the possible outcomes, consider the case of Alex Barlow, far more complex than that of Mr. Davidoff.

### A Dying Patient and the Issue of Scarce Resources: Alex Barlow's Case

Alex Barlow was a 19-year-old African American male who at 17 had been diagnosed with gliosarcoma (brain tumor) and given a life expectancy of less than one year. At the time of the bioethics consultation, Alex's care was being provided by the Pediatric Intensive Care Unit (PICU), although until this hospitalization he had been treated by an adult oncology service. His illness had recently entered a terminal phase despite an aggressive course of treatment involving surgery, radiation therapy, and chemotherapy. And despite these interventions, Alex continued to have headaches and seizures and had been frequently admitted to the hospital for care. Alex and his family repeatedly chose options of aggressive care and rejected any palliative care or hospice options presented to them. Alex continued to deteriorate and suffered from mild aphasia, memory loss, right-sided weakness, and gait problems that necessitated his using a four-sided cane.

Alex was able to participate in decisions about his care and communicate his preferences, which were consistently for aggressive care. Toward the end of his illness he appointed his sister as his health care proxy and his girlfriend as the alternate decider. At the time that a bioethics consultation was requested Alex was intubated, unconscious, and unresponsive, and had multiple organ failure. He had been in this state for approximately two months secondary to the effects of the brain tumor, sepsis, and a chronic lung infection.

Alex had experienced great sadness and dislocation in his life. As children, he and his sister had been abandoned by their biological mother and eventually had been adopted by an elderly foster care mother. When they were adolescents, their adoptive mother returned them to the foster care agency and revoked her adoption. Alex had been in juvenile detention for some parts of his adolescent years. Since age 16 he had been in touch with his biological mother and had had a constant girlfriend, who dropped out of college in the last year of his illness to care for him. His sister and his girlfriend were present nearly every day at the bedside and insisted that he responded to their presence. There was also an older man who frequently visited and was referred to as a brother.

There had been several confrontations between the care team and Alex's family (sister, girlfriend, and brother) as his health deteriorated. This conflict was not surprising, since the case was medically complex and the outcome increasingly grim. Moreover, Alex, like many other poor people and people of color without adequate health insurance coverage, had received episodic care from a series of institutions. Most recently, a phalanx of consultants had reiterated to the family that Alex was dying. That meeting had been a disaster and had led to bad feeling with all members of the family. At that point the social worker called for a bioethics consultation. In a brief memorandum about the case that she brought to the first meeting, she stated the ethical questions as follows:

1. What are the health care team's obligations to the well-being of Alex and to his protection from harm? What are its obligations to the family?
2. What are the health care team's obligations to provide Alex with medical care involving scarce resources when such care is deemed medically futile?
3. Should the health care team make decisions about Alex's care against the will of the health care proxy if they feel that it would prevent harm to Alex and prevent suffering?

As is the policy of the service, the bioethics mediator met first with the staff to try to understand the medical history and the present medical options. Members of the care team were concerned with Alex's continued stay in the PICU and with the administration of platelets, which were at that moment a scarce resource in the hospital. They did not know how to connect with the family around this dying patient and had failed, repeatedly, to reach an agreement about the course of Alex's care.

The mediator asked for a palliative care consultation before meeting with the family. Finally, the mediator, the social worker, the primary PICU attending physician, and the palliative care physician sat together with Alex's sister, girlfriend, and brother. The mediator opened the meeting by explaining that she was an employee of the hospital and that her task was to try to find some common ground where both the staff and the family could be comfortable with the plan of care for the patient. She explained that she did not come to make the decision but rather to help the parties understand each other better and reach some agreement. "Oh," the sister commented, "you're like a mediator."

The sister then embarked on a passionate presentation about her relationship with her brother and the course of his illness. She detailed the failures of all of the health care systems with which they had dealt. She attacked the various hospitals in which Alex had previously been treated and called attention to those times when they had not been adequately informed about the options and possible consequences of treatment. For example, she stated that they would not have agreed to the last chemotherapy if they had known that one consequence would be the need for blood and platelet transfusions. She emphasized that she and her brother were everything to each other and that she would never, under any circumstance, agree to any measure that would shorten his life by even a moment. He was the only person for all of her life who had been stable and loving. She was clear and powerful in her support of her brother and in her understanding of the system. She was extremely angry that some of the staff members talked in front of her brother as if he could not hear and did not tidy up the room adequately after changing his dressings and his diapers.

The mediator was impressed by the sister's intelligence, force, and advocacy and said so. She then commented that her task, in this case, was not only to listen and try to forge some common ground but also to place some constraints on the range of possible decisions. She explained the difference between "scarce" and "expensive" resources and identified platelets for transfusion as a scarce resource. She explained that scarce resources are distributed according to one of three general systems: first come, first served; lottery or random chance; and the judgment of the medical staff about which patient would be most likely to benefit from the transfusion. She explained all hospitals currently used the third option and that as long as there was a citywide shortage of platelets, this patient would not receive any, because there was no chance he would benefit.

The brother exploded. "Are you messing with my mind? Do you mean that my brother will not get this transfusion because you think that someone else will get better and he won't?" The mediator said yes, and the discussion about fairness and justice proceeded for some time. The family accepted that Alex would not be eligible to receive platelets. Finally, the sister said, "Thanks for telling us about the system. But, don't tell us that he is dying—we don't want to hear that. And don't tell us that you are moving him from the PICU."

The staff had discussed the possibility of moving Alex, and they were inclined to move him out of an intensive care bed since he could no longer benefit from that level of care. But the family had already been faced with one difficult decision, the mediator pointed out, and moving him from the PICU would totally isolate him and his family. Furthermore, the PICU had a few open beds at that moment and she believed the staff had obligations to the patient and to the family and that maintaining the patient in the unit fulfilled the obligations to the family. The staff, somewhat uncomfortably, agreed to maintain the patient in the unit. The mediator explained that if there were a catastrophe with multiple victims who needed the care of the unit, or a large number of very sick children arrived all at once at the hospital, the staff would again talk to the family about the location of the patient's care.

The mediator also brought up the family's anger that staff discussions indicating the patient was dying took place within his own room. The staff agreed to stop this practice, and the mediator recorded their agreement in the chart note.

Finally, the palliative care physician stated that he was going to suggest to the attending physician that she write a DNR order based on the narrow notion of "physiologic futility"—that there would be no way to restart the heart and lungs of this patient were he to go into cardiac arrest. The physician assumed the responsibility for making this decision and did not put the burden of the choice on the family. He described the state of the patient's lungs and the fragile nature of many of his systems. "The patient will not survive a resuscitation effort," he said, "because it will be too violent for his body to stand. He will die a violent death." The sister agreed that if his heart or lungs stopped that it would "be his time."

Was this a true mediation or was it just the imposition of the staff's will, through the supposedly neutral mediator, on the family? Alex's family stated its anger and dismay, heard finally why platelets would not be available to the patient, and accepted the DNR order that would smooth his death. They negotiated silence about his dying in the presence of the patient and attention to the state of his room. They were assured of his continued stay in the PICU unless needier patients arrived. They gained control of those elements of his care that they could influence and acknowledged those elements that were beyond their control. Perhaps they were comforted by the boundaries that had been set and to which they agreed. In any event, the relationships between the family members and the staff were far better after the mediation.

Alex Barlow's case highlights some critical themes in modern bioethics and contemporary American medicine. The family began this final set of interactions with the staff while the patient was dying. But this patient and family had been involved in a medical system that had failed to be faithful to them throughout the illness.

Also, they had been failed by the foster care system and enmeshed in the juvenile correctional system. Thus, they began, justifiably, with no sense of trust in the caregiver team and no inclination to accommodate this particular set of professionals. And the medical team was working at cross purposes. The primary attending physician was intent on moving the patient out of the PICU, which she felt needed to be open for newly admitted patients who could benefit from the high-tech care that it offered. The nurses were somewhat alienated by the behavior of the family and the palliative care team had not been sufficiently involved in the discussions with the family. All were decent and hard-working professionals involved in furthering a defensible set of goals but avoiding the sort of robust interactions with the family that the case required. The mediation provided the setting for the necessary discussions.

This case shows how a mediative approach by the bioethicist can repair relationships between caregivers and family members as they face the wrenching reality of an approaching death by making it possible not only for family members to speak but also to know they have been heard, while making clear the limits on care.

This chapter begins and ends with descriptions of bioethics mediations in which the use of the mediation process did not change the outcome in terms of what medical care would be given, but it did ensure that the concerns and needs of family members were identified, acknowledged, respected, and, to the extent that those needs did not violate legal or ethical norms, accommodated. The use of the mediation process allowed both families to begin to come to terms with their impending loss and restored communication and teamwork between the family and the health care team. How the process works is analyzed in detail in later chapters.

# 2

## *What Makes Bioethics Mediation Unique?*

THIS CHAPTER OUTLINES the unique factors that characterize bioethics mediations. Clearly, the institutional role of the bioethicist requires modification of some classical mediation practices. What is important, whether in classical mediation or in bioethics mediation, is that the mediator be aware, when deviating from the model, that he or she is doing so and why. Even more important, the mediator—in any setting—must make clear to all participants the "rules" under which he or she is operating.

There are several ways in which bioethics mediation differs from other types of mediation.

- The bioethics mediator is generally employed by the hospital.
- The bioethics mediator and members of the treatment team are repeat players.
- The bioethics mediator provides information, enforces norms, and ensures that resolutions fall within medical "best practice" guidelines.
- Deciding not to reach a resolution is not an option.
- The playing field is usually uneven for patients and their families.
- Confidentiality is limited to information not relevant to patient care.
- Time is of the essence.
- Bioethics mediations involve life-and-death issues.
- Facts play a different role.
- The person with the greatest stake in the dispute, the patient, is often not at the table.
- There may be a sequence of separate, prior meetings in addition to the group mediation.
- Bioethics mediations are almost always multiparty events.
- The parties usually do not sign an agreement to mediate.
- The physical setting may not be in the mediator's control.

- Bioethics mediators are often involved in following up on implementation of the agreement.
- All participants in a bioethics mediation have a common interest in the well-being of the patient.

## The Bioethics Mediator Is Generally Employed by the Hospital

In most classical mediation programs, the mediator is a neutral party with no allegiance to one side or the other. Either the parties agree on a mediator or a court or other agency assigns one. Mediators must reveal any prior contact with any of the participants, and any party who is uncomfortable having the mediation conducted by someone who already knows one of the other participants has the right to ask for a different mediator. In some programs, mediators are not allowed to handle cases in which they know the parties.[1]

In bioethics mediation, however, unlike in classical mediation, mediators are most often employed by the hospital. Their status as hospital employees means that bioethics mediators have the requisite substantive knowledge about the health care system, a knowledge of and commitment to the ethics of medicine, an understanding of the issues confronting patients and their families—and the caregivers—in acute care situations, and a base-line level of knowledge about issues of liability, as well as knowledge about the hospital hierarchy, practice, and personnel. Knowledge of the particulars and the history of staff can provide a crucial starting point for resolving conflicts, especially when events are constantly in flux and require speedy decisions.

When the first bioethics mediation programs were developed, as a practical matter, a stranger with no knowledge of the field, the staff personalities, and the institution would not have been given access to conflicts when life-and-death issues and legal liability were at stake. As caregivers become more familiar with mediation, some institutions may choose at times to use outside mediators, especially in cases where the level of distrust seems so high that an in-house mediator is unlikely to be effective. However, the urgent nature of most bioethics disputes makes it difficult, generally, for an outside mediator to be brought in quickly enough.

Whereas hospital bioethics consultants are not neutrals—independent persons with no previous connection to either side—they do come as new actors into a stale, and stalemated, context. They have no history with this patient and family.

---

1. This model of impartiality would not work in many other cultures where the only acceptable mediator would be one who knows both parties.

They are not responsible for the care decisions that produced no positive results or that resulted in a worsening of the patient's condition. They have not lost their tempers at moments of stress. They are not strangers but they are persons uninvolved in and neutral to this particular conflict. Furthermore, since hospital conflicts often involve life-and-death decisions, for which physicians, nurses, and the institution are legally and morally responsible, the health care providers may be more likely to trust mediators who are associated with the hospital to negotiate for consensus. Another benefit of the mediator's status as a hospital employee is that he or she is familiar with the clinicians and the prior patterns of the medical service involved. For example, if the mediator knows that a particular doctor has a principled objection to do not resuscitate orders and thus never writes them, the mediator will be better prepared to frame the discussion realistically with the patient and family if such an order is an issue. If the mediator confirms that the doctor's objection extends to a particular case, he or she can convene care providers to see whether the order may be ethically appropriate for this patient under these circumstances. Without this understanding of the doctor's values, the mediator may start the process at a less effective point.

There is a risk, however, that the patient or family may question the hospital-employee mediator's impartiality and assume that the mediator will take the side of the medical staff against them. Also, the medical staff may question the bioethics mediator's institutional loyalties. These concerns on both sides can compromise the mediator's position and make it difficult to build trust. But it is also true that successful mediations enhance the reputation of the mediators and make staff more likely to call for help in difficult situations.

## The Bioethics Mediator and Members of the Treatment Team Are Repeat Players

As mediation becomes more widely used to resolve disputes in the legal system and within large organizations, there is a risk that individual plaintiffs, employees, or consumers will be at a disadvantage at the mediation table when dealing with defendants who are familiar with the process and, perhaps, with the mediator. In many of those settings, however, the power imbalance created by having a repeat player at the table can be offset by the presence of an attorney or other advocate for the plaintiffs.

In bioethics mediation, the mediator and the medical team have often been involved in previous bioethics consultations or mediations and may have worked together in other professional contexts. Thus, the medical staff are familiar with the process and with the bioethics mediator and may have learned how to work the process (and spin the mediator) to achieve their goals. The family, however, is usually encountering both the mediator and the mediation process for the first time and is likely to feel that it does not have an advocate at its side. This is a problem to which mediators must be particularly attentive. An acknowledgment of the issue and the assurance that the patient and family will be supported may be required when beginning a mediation.

## The Bioethics Mediator Provides Information, Enforces Norms, and Ensures That Resolutions Fall within Medical "Best Practice" Guidelines

Constraints in the process that are set by legal rules and ethical principles are not unique to bioethics mediation. The mediator in a marital property dispute, for example, where the contesting parties seem to be working out a settlement that would leave one of them dependent on public assistance and the other one wealthy would be under an obligation to halt the mediation and explain that such a settlement would be counter to public policy and might constitute fraud. In addition to the boundaries established by law and public policy, bioethics mediation must operate within the boundaries of accepted medical practice, bioethics principles, relevant legal rules, and institutional policy.

But bioethics mediators have a much more direct and explicit responsibility, to transmit a body of knowledge about bioethics issues and enforce these norms. While they may use classical mediation process skills in the search for resolution, they also must be sure that any agreement is in the best interest of the patient, that it comports with the medical ethical norm of "do no harm," and that it meets the state's legal requirements. Furthermore, it is not sufficient for the mediator to arrive at a solution that all accept if that solution compromises the best widely accepted medical care plan and leaves the patient less well off. Later the patient or the family could sue for negligence, and the target of the suit would be the staff and the hospital, on whom legal responsibility falls. Thus the boundaries of a principled resolution are legal, ethical, and medical.

There is rich debate in the classical mediation community about whether the mediator should be responsible for ensuring that any agreement is fair or only for determining that the parties have the capacity to negotiate for themselves and, if so, helping them reach any agreement that works for them as long as it is not illegal (cf. Susskind 1981; Stulberg 1981; Bush 1989). Leonard Riskin (1984), for example, argues persuasively that mediators should be responsible for ensuring that agreements can meet three tests of fairness: Do the parties feel it is fair? Is it fair in terms of generally prevailing social norms? Is it fair to parties not at the table?

## Deciding Not to Reach a Resolution Is Not an Option

In many mediation contexts it is acceptable (even if not wise) to fail to reach an agreement. Litigants can continue to battle in the courts; neighbors can continue hostile relationships; parents and their teenager can continue to disagree about curfews. Stopping short of an agreement is rarely an option, however, in bioethics mediation. The welfare of the patient, standards of care, and legal requirements mean that decisions must be made about whether to continue or end treatment or about what treatment is to be provided. The attending physician and the institution are legally responsible for the care of the patient and must decide what measures are in the patient's best interest if negotiations fail. Thus, if agreement cannot be reached in the mediation session, a series of default rules for determining who makes decisions comes into play. The hospital personnel or, in some cases, a court may impose a solution consistent with their determinations of the best interests of the patient, the relevant decision-making rules, and the needs and interests of the institution.

## The Playing Field Is Usually Uneven for Patients and Their Families

In classical mediation, one of the mediator's jobs is to be alert for power imbalances that might prevent a fair negotiation of the issues. But as important as it is to recognize and address such problems, power imbalances are not an issue in most mediations.

In bioethics mediation there are almost always two predictable sources of power imbalance: disparity in knowledge and information and disparity in emotional status. The treatment team has far greater medical expertise and greater access to information than do most patients or family members. Even after the medical facts are presented, the bioethics mediator must constantly assess whether the patient or family understands the medical facts and is equipped to interpret the information, if not on an equal footing with all participants, at least sufficiently to make an informed decision.

Family members often respond with surprise to details about the case not because the information has not been presented to them but because they could not absorb it when they were told. On occasion, however, it may turn out that each member of the treatment team assumed that the others had relayed critical information or that some had communicated conflicting information. In addition, various family members may have heard information differently or assigned it different meanings. One of the roles of the bioethics mediator is to ensure that critical information is presented in such a way that the patient or the family members can hear it and absorb its meaning accurately.

Another way bioethics mediators overcome the imbalance and help families who must make difficult decisions for gravely ill or dying loved ones while also dealing with their own deep emotional distress is to slow down the discussion of the medical facts, ask the treatment team to explain medical terminology, and summarize without using euphemisms to mask unhappy prognoses.

There is a simple fact that goes some distance toward balancing this uneven playing field: in the medical context, and especially with complex and invasive treatments, the care process requires consent. If a patient—or the family of a decisionally incapacitated patient—refuses to consent to treatment, the provision of care is halted. Similarly, the vast majority of hospitals require consent from the patient or family to discontinue even futile treatment. Because of this requirement, the patient or family may be empowered at a particular juncture in the provision of care.

## Confidentiality Is Limited to Information Not Relevant to Patient Care

In bioethics mediation, the confidentiality that is a core principle of nonmedical mediation is limited. Good medical care requires that all providers share information about the patient's condition and care with each other across disciplines and between shifts. Documentation in the patient's chart is the means of accomplishing this information exchange and any treatment plan developed during mediation and new information significant to the patient's condition that comes out in mediation will be recorded in the patient's chart.

In addition, because of the fluid nature of bioethics mediations in which the mediator convenes as many of the caregivers as possible but may also need to speak with some people individually or with different groups by shift, who is and who is not a participant in the mediation process and therefore covered by any promise of confidentiality is often uncertain. It is therefore most fair and accurate to say that confidentiality, except for personal secrets unrelated to the care plan, is not guaranteed in bioethics mediation.

## Time Is of the Essence

Bioethics disputes arise, and must be resolved, in the context of evolving diagnoses and prognoses, with the punctuation of intermittent medical crises, in overcrowded diagnostic and surgical schedules, and framed always by therapeutic uncertainties.

Thus, unlike classical mediators who promise the parties that they will spend as much time as necessary or as much time as they want in mediation, bioethics mediators usually work under severe time pressures. They work on cases where medical conditions may be rapidly developing, where the need for a decision may be urgent, where at least one of the parties is often in an acute crisis, and in institutions where work demands on members of the treatment team may limit their participation. Thus, it can be tempting to rush through the meeting with the medical team when what is called for, and what will save time in the long run, is a slower pace that allows the participants to reach agreement on a plan for the meeting with the patient or family.

## Bioethics Mediations Involve Life-and-Death Issues

The stakes in classical mediation—custody of children, the future of a business, or protection of the environment—never involve life and death as they do in bioethics mediations. In some situations bioethics mediators may find that the extraordinary feelings of the participants in the face of serious illness or death are as important as—even more important than—the facts in a case.

## Facts Play a Different Role

Mediators in classical mediation are interested in facts only insofar as they give the mediator a sense of the nature and history of the problem or information that is useful in helping the parties shape a resolution.[2] It is often possible to resolve a

---

2. There is a subset of neutrals who, unlike the authors, believe that the mediation role includes evaluating the strengths and weaknesses of each side's case and predicting the likely outcomes in court. For them, deciding what the facts are does matter.

problem without reaching agreement about the facts. In bioethics mediation, however, it is essential that the parties involved in the decision understand and agree on
the medical facts—what is happening with the patient, the likely prognosis, and
how available treatments might affect the patient's condition—and that the patient and the family understand those medical facts. Not surprisingly, medical experts sometimes disagree about how data points (such as lab findings, test results,
or knowledge gained from physical exams) should be interpreted in establishing
medical facts. (For a more detailed discussion, see "Stage 3: Eliciting the Medical
Facts," p. 62.)

## The Person with the Greatest Stake in the Dispute, the Patient, Is Often Not at the Table

Many classical mediators require that all stakeholders and decision makers be present during the mediation, or, as a default option, if parties prefer to have an agent
represent them, be available by telephone for consultation. In bioethics mediation,
the patient's condition often precludes any meaningful participation. He or she
may be unable to participate in the mediation discussion and unable to be consulted about any agreement reached during the process.

   The voice of the patient should be heard, and in the patient's absence it can be
approximated by appeal to an advance directive that the patient completed before
incapacity intervened or by discussion with the family. Advance directives are of
two sorts, living wills and proxy designations, also called durable powers of attorney for health care decision making. These documents bring the patient's voice
forward to the discussion in real time. Living wills state specifically what the patient
would or would not want under various circumstances. But because the circumstance rarely fits the specifics, they are often irrelevant and thus easy to ignore.
Proxy appointments direct that health care decisions be made by a designated
person who is empowered to hear the medical facts, evaluate the alternatives, and
choose among them. The proxy appointment allows the designated person to negotiate interventions, which, as this book argues, reflects the realities of care.

   The major problem with advance directives, however, is that few patients have
them, particularly in the socioeconomic groups that use an inner city hospital.
Thus, it is much more common to elicit the patient's wishes by discussing him or
her with the family. The staff person, perhaps the bioethics mediator, perhaps a
nurse, physician, or social worker, tries to get the patient to be more than a phan-

tom at the table by asking questions about prior likes and dislikes and about reactions to medical care. This admittedly less-than-satisfying process reflects the reality that while ethical principles and the law are clear, the world of patients and their decisions is messy.

## There May Be a Sequence of Separate, Prior Meetings in Addition to the Group Mediation

In classical mediation, the norm is for the mediator and the parties to have limited contact before the beginning of the formal mediation. That preliminary contact might include discussions between the mediator and the parties or their representatives to determine whether mediation is the appropriate process or to decide who should be at the table. In addition, in complex cases, the participants may provide the mediator with confidential memoranda. But traditionally, discussion of the substance of the dispute is deferred until all participants meet with the mediator.

The practice for bioethics mediators is different. The bioethics mediator will usually choose to meet first with the members of the treatment team to try to reach agreement about the medical facts, the likely prognosis, the treatment options, and the recommended treatment. If agreement on any of these topics is not possible, the bioethics mediator will try to help the treatment team agree on how to present the different options and choices to the patient or patient's family members.

## Bioethics Mediations Are Almost Always Multiparty Events

Unlike the majority of classical mediations, bioethics mediation almost always involves more than two parties. Typically, several family members, physicians, nurses, and social workers, each with his or her own perception and interests, participate. And now, more and more, the participants may include a managed care representative (when a patient has reached the end of a reimbursed stay) and a member of the administrative staff, whose task is to limit the patient's length of stay.

Because most bioethics mediations have many participants, there are more opportunities for misunderstandings and miscommunications, and it may take more time to work through the process. For example, much of the resolution of the conflict may take place outside the joint mediation, in spontaneous meetings of some of the participants. Small caucuses that help different groups to understand the approach and attitude of others may help the process to move. (See Chapter 8.)

## The Parties Usually Do Not Sign an Agreement to Mediate

In classical mediation, mediators generally ask the parties to sign an agreement to mediate in order to provide for confidentiality of mediation communications, to make the "rules" of the process clear, and to encourage sharing of information. Participants' reactions to and questions about the contents of the agreement can provide the mediator with valuable information about their concerns. Moreover, the ritual value of signing can add to the idea that mediation is a serious enterprise.

In the bioethics mediation program on which this book is based, however, parties do not sign mediation agreements.[3] There are several reasons for not using an agreement in a bioethics case. First, most documents patients are asked to sign in the hospital setting are for the benefit of the institution, not the patient. Second, as discussed above, bioethics mediations are not truly confidential: in the hospital key decisions and discussions are recorded in the patient's medical chart, because good care depends on the ready accessibility of information about the patient. Third, families are under stress and distrustful and are likely to resist signing any agreements.

## The Physical Setting May Not Be in the Mediator's Control

In classical mediation, the mediator usually has some control over the physical setting in which the mediation takes place and can, at least, provide a place for everyone to sit and arrange the seating in a way that is likely to encourage discussion.[4] In the hospital setting, given the busy schedules of the members of the treatment team and work schedules of family members, it may be difficult to schedule mediation sessions in advance or find an appropriate meeting room. Initial sessions with the treatment team may take place leaning against a gurney in the hallway, in a corner of the nurses' station, or in a temporarily vacant patient room.

---

3. Some hospitals have elected to use outside mediators, who may choose to ask the participants to sign an agreement to mediate (Hyman 2002).

4. In some court-annexed programs, space is limited and mediators are forced to work in suboptimal settings, such as at tables in hallways.

## Bioethics Mediators Are Often Involved in Following Up on Implementation of the Agreement

In classical mediation, mediators may or may not be involved in ensuring that the agreed-upon solution is implemented. Most often, if one party to the agreement fails to act as expected, the dispute escalates to court. But in a hospital, unresolved conflicts are likely to return to the attention of the bioethics mediator. Even if a conflict has been resolved, the bioethics mediator will follow up with the nurses and doctors on the care team in an effort to maintain a close working relationship. It may also be necessary to "debrief" the team and allow them to review the conflict and reflect on their feelings about the outcome. Finally, established policies might need additions or corrections.

## All Participants in a Bioethics Mediation Have a Common Interest in the Well-Being of the Patient

The singular focus of all participants—on doing what is wanted by or is best for the patient—is unique to bioethics mediation.

# II

# A PRACTICAL GUIDE
# TO BIOETHICS MEDIATION

*This is the how-to part of the book. Here we discuss issues that should be considered in establishing a bioethics mediation program. Then we organize the process into stages and identify and illustrate the techniques of mediation. Following the steps outlined here is not, however, like following a recipe. The mediator must have the flexibility and sensitivity to know when to change the order of the steps and when to drop or combine steps. What is important for the mediator is to learn to recognize the stages so that he or she can call forth the appropriate techniques in support of a gradually emerging consensus.*

*Using the techniques of mediation provides some measure of control over situations that might seem too chaotic to approach, let alone resolve. If the bioethics mediator can refer to the stages of mediation and have some notion of the goals of each, it is possible to produce small gains in support of agreement that approaching the entire conflict head-on might not offer. As the cases in Part III illustrate, understanding the process may not always lead to a comfortable and unconflicted resolution but it allows the mediator to take on tasks with some confidence and work toward agreement.*

# 3

## *Before You Begin a Bioethics Mediation Program*

IN THIS CHAPTER we discuss the questions to consider before beginning a bio-ethics mediation program: what bioethics mediators need to know, the relative importance of substantive versus process skills, the pros and cons of institution-based mediators, the hospital staff best suited to conduct mediations, the value of co-mediation, the key roles for mediators, and the people who can initiate a mediation. This chapter provides a theoretical background for Chapter 4, which focuses on the stages of mediation, and Chapter 5, which focuses on techniques.

### What Bioethics Mediators Should Know

Mediating bioethics disputes demands knowledge of basic ethical and legal principles, as well as some understanding of medicine, the medical environment, and the culture of the particular institution. Mediators also should have an appreciation of the power imbalances between patients and their health care providers. Given the institutional realities, bioethics mediators, whether hospital employees or independent practitioners, must:

- be knowledgeable about the ethical principles and legal rules that frame the rights, duties, and obligations of patients, families, and the institution and that form the basis of bioethics analysis and the resolution of bioethics conflicts;
- be knowledgeable about the process of mediation, including having negotiation and conflict-management skills;
- be knowledgeable about the administrative and political workings of the particular institution (for example, who is the appropriate person or committee to contact if the care team cannot agree about the medical facts and the prognosis);[1] and

---

1. This sort of information is often acquired by independent mediators as part of core assessment and development before the mediation begins.

• be sufficiently knowledgeable about and experienced in health care to have a basis for asking appropriate questions about medical reality, alternative care plans, and options that might sharpen the issues, identify distinctions, or provide a platform for agreement.

The issue of the proper balance of process skills and substantive knowledge is the subject of ongoing debate in the mediation field. Most mediators would agree that the more technical the subject, the greater the importance of substantive knowledge.[2] On one hand, a mediator who is knowledgeable about the field, compared with one who lacks substantive knowledge, has more credibility in the minds of the parties and is better able to recognize common issues and concerns and to ask appropriate questions. Thus, he or she ultimately may be better able to help the parties reach a resolution. In the medical ethics context, where resolution is often urgent, this increased efficiency can be especially valuable. On the other hand, familiarity with a field and with its standard operating procedures may cause the mediator to make assumptions and fail to ask questions that intentionally or inadvertently challenge standard operating procedures but that might help the parties imagine new ways of doing things and lead to a better resolution.

### The Basic Ethical Principles

As noted in Chapter 1, bioethics rests on four central ethical principles: patient autonomy, beneficence, nonmaleficence, and distributive justice.

*Patient autonomy* is central to health care decision making. Respecting patient autonomy means giving priority to the values and wishes of the patient and thus supporting choices that are authentic and uncoerced. It confers a professional obligation to respect the patient's privacy and self-determination. When the patient is no longer able to participate in discussions and has executed an advance directive, that document, if it is a living will, or that person, if it is a proxy appointment, can guide the patient's care as he or she would have wanted. More often, however, there is no advance directive and then the care team and the family must muddle along together in an effort to figure out what the patient might have wanted and what is actually best for the patient.

Emphasis on patient autonomy is largely a Western phenomenon, informed by values of individualism and independence. Because reverence for autonomy is not

---

2. See p. 112, where the mediator's knowledge about reporting requirements for a death within 30 days after surgery helped her understand a surgeon's resistance to a do not resuscitate order.

universal, physicians should be sensitive to cultural differences that affect patients' comfort with notions of privacy, advance directives, and informed consent (see, e.g., Fadiman 1998). Furthermore, while it is legally and ethically appropriate to honor the wishes of the capable patient, physicians must also consider the ethical principles that give rise to other, often competing, obligations.

The principle of *beneficence* underlies obligations to provide the best care for the patient and balance the risks or burdens of care against the benefits. Beneficence often involves prolongation of life, restoration of function, relief from pain and suffering, and protection from harm. Beneficence resonates most with caregivers, whose mission is to provide therapeutic benefit and shelter from harm. Notions of nurturing and protecting reach their fullest expression in caring for those who are the most vulnerable. However, perceptions of benefit and best interest are not purely scientific; they involve expectations, goals, and value judgments. Recognition that patients and their physicians may differ in these assessments is at least partly responsible for the noticeable shift from physician paternalism to greater emphasis on patient choice.

At the very core of the healing professions is the principle of *nonmaleficence*, captured in the ancient maxim, "First, do no harm." This principle grounds obligations to avoid the intentional infliction of harm or suffering. Most, if not all, therapies carry the potential for some risk as well as benefit, and it would not be feasible to limit the therapeutic arsenal to treatments that are entirely benign. Nevertheless, the benefits of recommended treatments are expected to outweigh the possible harms, and physicians are required to discuss that calculus with their patients.

*Distributive justice* refers to those principles of social cooperation that define what each person in the society is due or owed—in short, what is fair. The several types of justice all share the basic formal notion of treating similar cases similarly. Distributive justice, the form of justice most relevant to medical ethics, concerns the norms and standards for allocating benefits and burdens across a given population. Distributive justice demands that the benefits, risks, and costs of actions— in medicine, access to resources related to physical and mental health—be apportioned fairly and without discrimination.

Society must confront such questions as, Is it fair to allocate organs for transplant on the basis of the patient's ability to pay? Is it fair for health insurance plans to provide more generous coverage for the treatment of physical illnesses than for the treatment of mental illnesses? According to the principle of distributive justice, there should be ethically defensible reasons why certain individuals or groups of individuals receive benefits or endure burdens that other individuals or groups do not.

Many scholars have noted that the fourth principle is distinct from the first three. Whereas the first three have found their way into common medical practice and discourse, the principle of distributive justice has been honored more in the breach than in the observance. A country that fails to provide universal access to health care, for example, has not taken the idea of justice very seriously (Beauchamp and Childress 1994).

### Principles of Negotiation

A significant part of the mediator's role is to facilitate a negotiation.[3] Fisher and Ury (1981, chs. 2–6), in their groundbreaking work *Getting to Yes*, suggest five guidelines for productive, problem-solving negotiation.

- Separate the people from the problem.
- Focus on interests, not positions.
- Generate options for mutual gain.
- Use objective criteria.
- Know your BATNA (best alternative to a negotiated agreement).

Fisher and Ury (1981, 17–40) point out that too often egos and personalities become the focus of a negotiation, with the result that the negotiators neglect the problem. Thus, many negotiations get no further than an exchange of positions— You must pay me $X; I won't pay more than $Y—and never get to the point of developing ways to satisfy the interests represented by the positions (41–57). Often negotiators get stuck by focusing only on the first ideas for addressing the problem rather than taking time to develop a range of options and then evaluating the benefits and drawbacks of each (58–83). Most important, Fisher and Ury (1981, 101–11) teach that while negotiators may be able to improve their BATNA's and therefore improve their negotiating positions, they should not walk away from an offer that is better than their best nonagreement option.

More recent scholars have described the negotiator's task as balancing the tension between creating and claiming value (Lax and Sebenius 1986, 29–45; Mnookin, Peppet, and Tulumello 2000, 11–43), empathy and assertiveness (Mnookin, Peppet, and Tulumello 2000, 44–68), and principals and agents (Mnookin, Peppet,

---

3. For a detailed discussion of negotiation theory, see Lax and Sebenius 1986; Mnookin, Peppet, and Tulumello 2000; Arrow et al. 1995; and Shell 1999.

and Tulumello 2000, 69–91). Skilled negotiators must both assert their own interests and demonstrate that they understand the interests of the other side. Negotiators also must be aware of the tensions in the principal-agent relationship. For example, the interest of a client in keeping home-decorating costs down may be at odds with the interest of the decorator whose compensation is based on a percentage of all purchases. In the health care setting, the patient and family may desire expensive cutting-edge treatments while the hospital or managed care insurance company may resist as a cost-limiting measure.

### Ways People Respond to Conflict

As conflict managers, mediators should be aware of and comfortable with the wide variety of ways people respond to conflict, recognizing that all responses are "normal." People involved in conflict may become loud and exaggerate their grievance or they may shut down and express themselves in a guarded manner. Some may even deny that there is a conflict.[4] People involved in conflict experience a variety of physiological symptoms—a knot in the stomach, flushing, sweating, racing heart. They may become suspicious, hostile, confused, defensive, pessimistic, and less trusting. Perhaps most important, people in conflict stop listening to each other.

Conflict tends to be expressed by the parties through positions, insults, generalities, and threats (Shaw 2000). The mediator's job is to help the parties refocus so that they can discuss their interests, communicate productively, focus on the issues that should be resolved, generate options, and evaluate proposals for resolution.

Introducing a third person into a conflict changes the dynamics. The disputing parties must explain the nature of the conflict, their perspective on its sources, and their idea of the correct solution. They usually want to look good to the mediator, and so they may become more rational and less extreme in the way they express themselves or in the demands they make on the other party. Or they may feel it is safe to express previously suppressed strong emotions. The parties may also distrust or question the fairness or neutrality of the mediator. They may have the same response as spatting children when a parent enters the room, each seeking to win over the neutral party and demonstrate that he or she is in the right, that the other is in the wrong and at fault.

---

4. Many people think it is unprofessional or unseemly to be in a conflict and shy away from using that term to describe the problem that brings them to mediation; see pp. xv–xvi.

## Who Should Conduct Bioethics Mediations
### *In-House versus Independent Mediators*

As pointed out in Chapter 2, there is considerable difference of opinion about who is best suited to conduct mediations in a hospital setting: a hospital staff person steeped in the process, procedures, assumptions, and philosophy of the institution or an independent, noninstitutionally based mediator. Certainly the in-house mediator will have private knowledge of the quirks and peculiarities of the institution, as well as the personalities and preferences of the medical staff, though it could be argued that this insider knowledge can be acquired with a few well-placed early questions. The in-house person will be more efficient at the outset; more comfortable with the participants and the setting; more knowledgeable about the power politics and political camps; and able to write a chart note in the chart, alerting the rest of the care team to the discussions and the outcome, a critical ability (see box). Furthermore, the fact that the mediator is part of the institution provides reassurance to the health care providers that he or she understands the complexities of the setting and the needs of the participants. This understanding provides an effective foundation for building trust. In some situations, however, nonhospital mediators, despite their being unable to write a chart note, might be preferable. Because outsiders are free of the institution's politics and power structure, outsiders' impartiality would not be questioned and therefore they might find it easier to gain the trust of the participants.

Most hospitals so far seem to have used in-house bioethics mediators, preferring their knowledge of institutional mores and the health care system and bioethical and legal principles, as well as their ease of access to staff, even though this choice may mean some diminution of neutrality, or at least the appearance of neutrality. To repeat, hospitals are reluctant to import an unknown person into the intellectually complex, legally paranoid, risk-aversive, regulation-defensive world of acute-care medicine. As it is, hospital administrators are continually worried about negative publicity and litigious patients. The more savvy, or the more suspicious and distrustful, administrators report that malpractice attorneys regularly prowl the halls for potential cases or have staff members in their employ to identify discontented patients and families. This is not fertile ground for the intervention of an unknown person into the management of a complex, controversial case. Until physicians, hospital administrators, and other caregivers become familiar enough with mediation to understand that the mediator does not impose resolution on the parties, they may be reluctant to use external mediators. Nonetheless, some hospitals

---

## The Importance of the Chart Note

The chart note communicates the salient characteristics of the bioethics dispute and whether it has been resolved, and if so, how it has been resolved. The chart note is important to the process of care. As shifts change, new staff must be able to understand whether the dispute remains and where the parties stand. If a resolution has been reached, the health care team needs to know the terms and conditions of the agreement. The chart note is the only effective and certain way to communicate all the critical pieces of information about a case among and between the teams and professionals. The chart is a legal document defining the reality of care. By law, only hospital personnel can write in it. Until this law is changed, the effectiveness of the noninstitutional mediator is limited. However, institutional administrators could certainly approve of a note written by a mediator about a conflict and place it in the chart. See p. 78 for a sample chart note.

---

have turned to outside mediators knowledgeable about bioethics and the health care system to intervene in bioethical disputes.[5]

It is a commonplace in epidemiological discussions to note that two anecdotes do not equal data. Nonetheless, the recent experience of a team of mediators, both attorneys, both knowledgeable about medicine, who were hired by medical institutions to mediate particularly difficult cases that had pitted patient, family, and care team against each other provides preliminary support for the benefits of hiring independent mediators in bioethics disputes. Both the mediators and the institution were comfortable with the arrangement (Hyman 2002). Further studies are needed, however, on the relative merits of the in-house and the independent mediator.

### Hospital Staff

In general, the strategy that has worked best in bioethics mediation has been to teach the process of mediation to professionals who are already knowledgeable about bioethics. A consideration of who might be the most appropriate staff to train to mediate bioethics disputes should, for example, include nurses. Their consistent involvement in patient care and their understanding of the day-to-day de-

---

5. Chris Stern Hyman and Marc Fleischer, principals in Medical Mediations Groups, have been brought in to mediate some hospital bioethical disputes (Hyman 2002).

tails of care make them excellent candidates, though in many institutions nurses are not in positions of power and therefore might, at least initially, lack credibility with physicians. Increasingly, however, nurse practitioners and nurse administrators are assuming greater responsibilities for patient care and thus are more likely now to be accepted as mediators by their physician colleagues. Furthermore, recently trained physicians are more accustomed to collaborative practice. As with all emerging and evolving solutions, the creation of nurse bioethics mediators will likely be more fitting in some hospitals than in others. Both the process and the professions will have to find their way. Physicians willing to spend the time necessary to be trained as mediators and to conduct mediations, social workers, clergy, and psychologists should also be considered as potential bioethics mediators.

There are some within the hospital structure who are generally not good candidates to become bioethics mediators. Risk managers and hospital attorneys who have responsibility for possible future litigation, for example, have very particular roles in health care institutions, primarily representing the hospital and protecting it from possible future liability.[6] Their role as authoritative decision makers should it be impossible to reach an agreement in mediation will generally make them inappropriate bioethics mediators. Even though hospital attorneys and risk managers are not good candidates to conduct bioethics mediations, they may find it useful to participate in mediation training in order to understand the process and therefore be in a better position to direct developing disputes to mediation and to participate effectively in the process.

Consider the following example. A patient's family wishes him to remain in the hospital, rather than be transferred to a nursing home, despite the fact that the staff have concluded that he no longer requires treatment in an acute care setting. The family believes that the care in the hospital is superior and more likely to prolong the patient's life; in addition, the nursing home is quite distant, which would make family visits very difficult. In the staff's view, the patient's continued presence is a misuse of resources, depriving other patients of needed attention and creating a financial drain on the hospital, which is no longer being fully reimbursed for the bed. The hospital counsel's function in this case is to assist in the removal of the patient from the hospital as quickly as possible, using court intervention if necessary. It is possible that the attorney might try to negotiate a compromise, using some of the same skills as would a mediator, since litigation is expensive and a potential

---

6. In other settings attorneys make excellent mediators.

exists for negative publicity. This compromise might resemble the same arrangement that a mediator would encourage the parties to agree to on their own, but the attorney must make it clear to the family that he or she represents the interests of the hospital in this process.

Consider also a dispute that arises between a patient's internist and the director of the surgical intensive care unit where the patient is currently being treated. The internist believes the patient should be removed from life support; the surgeon is opposed. In this situation, the function of the hospital attorney is to determine the relative legal authority in support of each side's position. If the law supports the internist (e.g., the patient has left an advance directive covering these circumstances), the surgeon will be instructed to honor that request or transfer the patient to another treating physician; if he or she refuses, senior administration will be asked to intervene. Although mediation skills may be important in managing this particular dispute, the hospital attorney's role in most instances is more analogous to that of an arbitrator or judge than to that of a mediator.

### Ethics Committees versus Consultants

Some ethics committees are clearly skilled, committed, interested, and courageous. But some are controlled by administrative forces in the institutions and have neither independence nor intellectual mettle. Moreover, mediation by committee would require training all of the committee members and then arranging them in such a way as to not overwhelm the other participants. The first requirement seems unlikely and the second impossible.[7]

### Co-mediation versus the Single Mediator

The co-mediation model doubles the chance that all important information will be heard, interests will be identified, and issues will be framed in a way that lets all participants hear what is being said.[8] In bioethics mediation, where issues are complex, feelings are intense, and there often are a large number of players, co-mediation is the preferred model (for a situation in which co-mediation was invaluable, see Chapter 8). Unfortunately, the reality of limited resources means that most bioethics mediators work alone.

---

7.  Ross et al. (1993) note that mediation may be one of the tasks of an ethics committee but the authors do little to support the idea, pointing out that committees vary widely and some have almost no authority or importance within their institutions.

8.  For a more detailed discussion of co-mediation, see Love and Stulberg 1996.

## Who Can Request a Bioethics Mediation and Who Must Participate

Traditional clinical medical consultation takes place when the attending physician requests the diagnostic or therapeutic judgment of a colleague, usually from a list of experts in a particular subspecialty. In contrast, bioethics consultation requests should be permitted to come not only from the attending physician but from nurses, social workers, and other members of the team, a family member, or the patient. The consultant who is invited by someone other than the attending physician fits into the evolving pattern of consultants in the modern hospital setting. As hospitals become more concerned with issues of cost, quality, safety, and patient satisfaction, they are less constrained by the notion of the attending physician as the unquestioned, final authority. The notion of the "uninvited consultant" (Blustein, Post, and Dubler 2002, 47–56) is becoming more common in medicine. The engine of consensus is a powerful one that can pull the care plan in new directions. Despite the initial nonparticipation in bioethics mediations of some of the players, even including, in very rare instances, the attending physician, as the discussion goes on, all concerned usually join in. When they do not, clearly, the attending physician must agree, finally, to implement the plan; grudging agreement will be as effective for this purpose as enthusiastic support. In this sort of case, the consultant assumes the role of "advocate for the consensus." One caveat, however: if someone other than the attending physician calls the consult, the first step of the mediator is to contact the attending physician and, if possible, secure his or her cooperation.

# 4

## The Stages of Bioethics Mediation

THIS CHAPTER PRESENTS a brief introduction to the stages of a typical bioethics mediation, mediator activity at each stage, and how mediator skills can be helpful in dealing with bioethics problems. Its purpose is to describe the mediation process and show what mediators do to make the process work.

### Overview of the Stages of Bioethics Mediation

Mediative bioethics intervention is a fluid process. To provide structure for discussion and training we have divided the process somewhat artificially into seven stages.[1] Be warned, however: in real life events never proceed in a predictable and orderly manner. The seven stages of a bioethics mediation are:

- Stage 1: Assessment and preparation
- Stage 2: Beginning the mediation
- Stage 3: Presenting and refining the medical facts
- Stage 4: Gathering information
- Stage 5: Problem solving
- Stage 6: Resolution
- Stage 7: Follow-up

Stages 1–7 represent a melding of traditional ways of describing mediation as a process that takes place in stages (Moore 1996, 66–67) and an analysis of what happens in actual bioethics mediations. Although the activities described within each stage may appear to be distinct and sequential, most mediations are far from linear.[2] They tend to move through various phases in which each party may be at a different stage. For example, some participants may be ready to start problem solving

---

1. The stages describe what typically occurs during bioethics mediation when the mediator is an employee of the hospital. The entry activities an external mediator would need are not discussed here.

2. For an attempt to describe mediation in a non-linear manner, see Della Noce 2001.

while others are still intent on making certain their views of the situation have been heard. Moreover, participants often circle back to earlier stages of the process, especially as they near the time when they must make difficult decisions. Similarly, the mediator may take steps throughout the process that are described here as characteristic of one particular stage. Our purpose in this chapter is to provide a step-by-step guide for mediators that includes suggestions about where they may want to make changes and enough theory to guide the variations. In any particular case, steps might occur in a different order and some steps might be eliminated entirely. Interventions that are critical in one case might be counterproductive in another. The reader's focus should be on understanding the goals of each stage and the techniques that can best be used to accomplish each goal.

Throughout the process, mediators play multiple roles: convener, amplifier, coach, guide, process manager, information gatherer, referee, seeker of common interests, facilitator, reality tester, and empathizer. Bioethics mediators have the additional roles of norm enforcers and staff educators.

During all stages of a bioethics mediation the mediator has certain overriding obligations that arise from the intimidating nature of the medical setting and the tremendous imbalance of power and education that separates patients and families from staff. The mediator must manage the negotiation; prevent the staff from "ganging up" on the patient and the family; ensure that family members, increasingly supported by legal counsel who may be intimidating to the medical team, do not distort the medical realities and possibilities; and provide the "neutral space" that permits a principled resolution to emerge. Throughout the process, the mediator maintains an impartial stance by having no investment in any specific outcome, by facilitating the discussion among all of the parties, by identifying the sources of the conflict, and by maximizing the options for resolution.

Although bioethics mediation works within a legal framework and the bioethics mediator does provide information about the governing legal rules (see below, Jennifer's Case), it is not useful for the bioethicist, when in the role of mediator rather than consultant, to offer complicated legal analysis. In those rare situations in which detailed legal analysis is required, a legal expert can be invited to participate or to counsel one of the parties outside of the mediation or to make a presentation during a subsequent mediation session. Likewise, the bioethics mediator should not offer therapeutic counseling. Again, experts can be used for this purpose but it is important for the parties not to confuse the role of the mediator with that of other experts. The following case illustrates some of the difficult issues typical of bioethics mediations.

### How Does the Process Work? Jennifer's Case

Jennifer was an 18-year-old patient who had been hospitalized many times for complications arising from Von Recklinghausen's ("Elephant Man") disease. This disease causes huge and unsightly tumors all over the body, internally and externally. Not only is the condition disfiguring but it interferes with the function of various organ systems and is often life-threatening.

This particular hospital admission was made necessary by the growth of a tumor that had developed on Jennifer's neck, closing off the trachea and preventing her from breathing without mechanical support. She had entered the hospital and been put on a ventilator immediately to prevent suffocation. Diagnostic tests determined that it would be possible to remove enough of the tumor surgically to enable her to breathe on her own. However, discussions with Jennifer indicated that she did not want the surgery, despite its promise of relief. Carefully communicating by pad and pencil, she explained that she had suffered enough with the disease and wanted to reject the surgery. She realized that the result of her refusal would be death.

Her attending physician in the intensive care unit wrote the following note in the chart: "Patient is an adult and is capable of choosing the kind of care she wants. She should be removed from the intensive care unit and placed in a private room to die. Morphine should be provided when needed."

The primary care physician called for a bioethics consult, stating, "I don't see any difference between this action and that of Dr. Kevorkian. How can we do this and help her to die? Isn't that assisting in a suicide?"

The bioethics consultant convened all of the parties for a formal mediation. In addition to Jennifer (who had requested that her parents not be present) and the two physicians, the meeting included the primary nurse, the social worker, the pain specialist, and a member of the liaison psychiatry service. The psychiatrist was invited at the suggestion of the mediator, who felt that a formal evaluation of Jennifer's decisional capacity might be useful for the upcoming mediation.

The bioethics consultant, acting in the role of mediator, began the meeting by describing the telephone call that she had received the day before and her sense that all of the involved care providers ought to meet. The primary care physician reviewed Jennifer's history and present condition and renewed his argument that letting Jennifer die was assisted suicide. Jennifer's intensive care unit physician reported that Jennifer had stated that she had suffered enough and was no longer interested in living under these conditions, a position that seemed to him eminently rational. The liaison psychiatrist, supported by the nursing staff, indicated that Jennifer was lucid and very knowledgeable about her condition and was neither clinically depressed nor suicidal. She had, in fact, considered the alternatives and had decided that the pain and anguish of surgery, which would likely remove the immediate threat of death but would still leave her in a great deal of pain, extremely disabled, and very disfigured, were not worth the gain in extra days, weeks, or even months of life.

The social worker explained that Jennifer's parents had been present at all of the conversations and were in agreement with their daughter, as was her priest. The mediator explained that historically both medical ethicists and the courts had distinguished between suicide, characterized by the intent and the inception of an act designed to bring about death, and a refusal of care that, as in Jennifer's case, might lead to death. In the latter case, the patient is not choosing death (most patients, even those who refuse care, do not want to die) but rejecting the pain and suffering of the intervention. The mediator pointed out that this right of a decisionally capable patient to refuse care in the face of life-threatening illness is grounded in the common-law right of self-determination and in the right of liberty protected by the Fourteenth Amendment to the U.S. Constitution. It is also grounded in the philosophical notion of autonomy.

The mediator further distinguished the acts of Dr. Jack Kevorkian, whose patients would not have died from an underlying condition by refusing care. For these patients, only an aggressive intervention to interrupt functioning organ systems could bring about death. The staff seemed comfortable with this explanation but were still uncomfortable with the order to "move her to another room and let her die." The nurses, in particular, were distressed by the notion that Jennifer would die, when her condition, at least in the short run, was remediable.

The mediator then asked what possible scenarios existed for Jennifer once the ventilator tube had been withdrawn. The discussion produced a range of care options, all focused on the use of morphine, and uncovered the providers' fears that the appropriate use of the drug might hasten Jennifer's death. In addition the nurses were particularly concerned that Jennifer would die alone, away from the staff whom she knew and was comfortable with. The primary care physician remained leery of "causing" death.

In response to the concerns of the nursing staff, the mediator asked for a meeting with just that staff. In the meeting, the nurses first stated that their ethic of care required that they care for Jennifer according to standard protocols that supported life and not death. But, the mediator argued, this is a dying patient; there was nothing they could do to change the outcome.

Further discussion revealed that the nurses felt that their real obligation was to show respect and give comfort, and their core commitment was to staying with Jennifer so that she would not be alone and abandoned during her dying hours.

The mediator reconvened the larger group and suggested that a consensus on a care plan had been reached. Since the death would likely be quite speedy and would therefore not amount to an unjust squandering of scarce resources, Jennifer could be permitted to remain in the intensive care unit until she died, with continued staff support from the people she had known. The mediator further commented that the U.S. Supreme Court has held, in an opinion on physician-assisted suicide, that the provision of adequate pain control, even if it hastens death, is not a violation of law and that both the American Nursing Association and the American Medical Association have ethics opinions on record stating that the secondary effect of hastening death should not be a barrier to the necessary and effective use of pain medication. This opinion, she stated, in continuing her education of staff, was also supported by the bioethics and the religious literature. Finally, she reminded staff of a recent article in which polled medical staff agreed that the single greatest abuse of patients is the inappropriate withholding of pain control at the end of life. The ethical issue, she suggested, would be generated by withholding effective pain control, not by providing adequate analgesia.

The staff talked about their commitment to this patient and their feelings of failure and frustration at her impending death. Not everyone was totally comfortable with the conclusion reached. Some of the nurses still felt that they wanted to try one last time to persuade Jennifer to undergo surgery, and one of the nurses did engage in this effort, although gently. All felt, however, that they could accept Jennifer's final decision. The mediation closed with agreement on a care plan that would permit Jennifer to remain in the intensive care unit until her death and would ensure that she received sufficient morphine to relieve her discomfort during the dying process.

## Stage 1: Assessment and Preparation

### Assessing the Situation

*Receiving the consultation request.*   The bioethicist may receive an official request for a consult or hear informally about a dispute and take the initiative to ask those involved whether a consult might be helpful. An official request might come from an intern or resident, an attending physician, a subspecialty fellow, a nurse, a social worker, a patient, a family member, or occasionally, an administrator. The bioethicist's first task is to assess the situation to get a preliminary sense of what intellectual, medical, ethical, emotional, and dynamic issues are involved and to determine whether the case is appropriate for mediation.

*Evaluating the nature of the dispute.*    The initial evaluation of the dispute is likely to require making some telephone calls to members of the health care team, reviewing the chart, and quickly convening a meeting of the involved members of the care team. The bioethics mediator should identify the patient, elicit a preliminary notion of the patient's decisional capacity (or at least identify whether capacity is at issue), determine the existence or nonexistence of family and the family's level of involvement, and explore the disputed issue as perceived by the referring staff member.

Having taken these preliminary steps, the mediator should attempt to determine what is generating the conflict.[3] Is it the personal philosophy of one of the caregivers (most likely, one of the physicians) or the personal philosophy or deeply held religious beliefs of the patient or family? Often the origin of the dispute is the difficulty the family is having coming to terms with the impending death of a loved one. Another common cause of disputes is inadequate communication or conflicting communication among members of the team but more often between the health care providers and patient or family members. Care providers may give mixed messages about the patient's condition or prognoses, assuming that someone else will take responsibility for delivering painful information.[4]

*Gathering information about the medical facts.*    Before the actual mediation takes place, the mediator should begin to establish the "medical facts." These include consensus agreements among the staff about the meaning of the medical narrative, the present data, and the observations of staff regarding the patient's improvement or deterioration. For the purposes of mediation, a medical fact is an interpreta-

---

3. From here on, for simplicity, we refer to the bioethics mediator as "the mediator."

4. If it is determined after a full mediative process that the physician's personal code of ethics precludes his or her participation in a medical activity that has been suggested (at issue might be discontinuation of ventilator support) and if the care plan is otherwise ethically and legally permissible, the mediator might take on the role of bioethics consultant and suggest that the physician resign from the case. Were the physician to refuse to resign, the mediator as bioethics consultant might need to refer the matter for resolution by a higher administrative authority.

tion of data at a particular moment that considers the patient in the light of the overall history of the illness. Medical facts have the ring of scientific objectivity, but determining what counts as a medical fact is a matter of selection and interpretation, and that process reflects normative assumptions.

Establishing the medical facts requires as much of a process as constructing an intervention plan. It often involves, at minimum, reviewing the chart, speaking to individual members of the treatment team, and facilitating a discussion of the patient's condition at a meeting of all involved medical staff (see below, "Meeting with the care team"). If, as is usual in bioethics mediations, the mediator chooses to meet separately with the care team and also to have an initial meeting with the patient or family, he or she should explain the reasons to both, label the separate meetings as the start of the mediating or conflict resolution process, and alert all participants to the need to meet together as soon as possible to begin to talk face-to-face about the resolution.

Issues of hierarchical standing among and within departments in the medical center come into play in this step. In the attempt to establish the medical facts, the mediator must try to understand the underlying tensions among the staff and the dynamics of the particular medical service. Most medical centers shelter a series of separate freestanding fiefdoms, all with particular histories and working styles that affect how the "facts of the case" will be established. And who arrives at the facts makes a difference as well. The patient's current condition may appear in one way when the attending physician or various consultants review the tests and laboratory values and quite another when the nurses are surveyed. Patients whose laboratory values seem to be improving may nonetheless look to experienced nurses as though they have begun dying.

*Establishing the decision history of the case.*    This is a particularly important step if the conflict has been going on for some time. Mature cases often involve a patient transferred from long-term care or one for whom discharge planning has been especially difficult or who has had a difficult and lengthy course of care in this hospital or in another acute care institution.

For example, if a patient has been seen for dialysis at one hospital where he was disruptive and difficult to manage and for some reason he arrives at a new hospital, the attempts of this new institution to discharge the patient back to his previous site are likely to be unproductive. Any mediator who disregards this history is likely to be consumed by the multi-institutional interests in avoiding problem patients.

*Meeting with the care team.*    A preliminary meeting with the medical staff is essential to understanding the history and present condition of the patient and a necessary precondition to discussing the medical and ethical options with the patient and family. Conflict between staff and the patient or family may be the result of discussions with consultants or of discussions with friends or relatives who practice medicine in other settings.

At this first meeting of the care team the mediator should take the following steps:

- Ask the attending physician (or, in a teaching hospital, the intern), primary nurse, and most involved social worker to present the case.
- Identify the parties to the conflict from among the staff.
- Begin to gather data on whether the patient is perceived as decisionally capable, whether there are any advance directives, or whether a surrogate decision-making process is contemplated.
- If family members are involved, determine who has been most involved until the time of the consult.
- If no family members are involved, and if the patient is not decisionally capable, determine whether the institution has special provisions for identifying the interests and protecting the rights of incapacitated patients who are without surrogates.

While there is no controversy about whether and when this meeting should take place, in some nonacademic institutions with attending physicians whose presence on the hospital premises is only sporadic, it may be difficult to schedule a time for all of the medical staff to meet. Nonetheless, the task of establishing the medical facts is so critical to the next stages of the process, and to any intelligent discussion with the patient and family, that the mediator should expend substantial efforts in pursuit of this initial caregiver meeting. If it is impossible to convene the team, it may suffice to hold separate conversations with different members of the team, repeating to each, with permission, the comments of his or her colleagues. This is a poor second, however, since clarity about the diagnosis and prognosis is most likely to emerge in the give and take of professional observations in a face-to-face meeting.

During the meeting with the medical team the mediator will try to reach agreement about the medical facts, the treatment options, the likely prognosis, and the recommended treatment. If agreement on any of these topics is not possible, the mediator will try to help the treatment team agree on how to present the differences and choices to the patient or patient's family members. In some situations—if the patient or the family members are already aware of the differences or if the mediator thinks that participation by the family members will keep the focus on the common interest in the patient's well-being—the mediator might decide to have the patient or the patient's family members present from the beginning. But more often the mediator will meet first with the treatment team.

Once the mediator has helped the medical staff reach consensus about what will be said and how the issues will be presented—even if they do not agree on the treatment implications—the mediator needs to anticipate issues that might develop as the discussion with the patient unfolds, what questions the patient is likely to ask or want to ask but be timid about raising, and what additional information or support systems need to be available for the patient or family in order to make it possible for them to make a decision.

*Meeting the patient and family.*    The mediator, either before or just after meeting with the care team, should introduce himself or herself to the patient or patient's family, or both, evaluate whether decisional capacity is an issue, learn the patient's history, and assess the family's priorities. At a minimum, the mediator informs the patient and the family about the request for a bioethics consultation.

*Assessing the time constraints.*    Timely intervention is critical to the success of many bioethics mediations. If one of the treatment options requires an immediate decision in order to preclude some medical catastrophe, the usual process of mediation might be truncated by the demand of the intervention. In addition, unattended disagreements tend to fester and worsen. Staff, family members, and patients settle into hardened positions that make movement difficult.

In most cases, however, even in acute care settings, time will not be so constricted as to warp the process. The mediator should also keep in mind that time is often the ally of an ethically comfortable plan. A preliminary consensus can be reached, for example, if it includes an agreement to reassess the situation in 24 or 48 hours. If the medical situation does not require an immediate plan, time will often work to support agreement. In the increasingly cost-conscious world of acute care medicine, however, where shortening the aggregate "length of stay" determines fiscal integrity, time is an increasingly scarce commodity.

*Identifying areas of uncertainty and gathering more pre-mediation information.* In cases where the medical staff disagree fundamentally on the likely prognosis, the mediator might, before convening the initial mediation session with the patient, family, and health care team, take additional action to help reach consensus or clarify the disagreement. Interventions that might be helpful include:

- Assembling the bioethics committee, or a subset of the committee, to see whether new players in a multidisciplinary setting can open new avenues of questioning and agreement
- Involving the medical director or some other medical or administrative authority who might convene all of the parties and direct the discussion more forcefully toward a consensus; as a variant, the mediator might ask that the case be referred to a committee within the institution, which would be empowered to arrive at a working set of facts for the case (both of these solutions demonstrate, arguably, the failure of the mediative process, but the obligation of the mediator to reach a timely solution may demand such immediate action in order to facilitate the rest of the process)
- Asking for the patient to be presented as the basis for discussion by the full divisional or departmental staff, if the relevant service has regularly scheduled rounds or conferences
- Asking for a literature search to enrich the discussion

These initial stages of the mediation process vary enormously in their intellectual and administrative complexity. Many mediators simply bring the staff together or arrange a meeting among the staff, the patient, and the family and thus facilitate the identification and resolution of disagreements. Only the most difficult cases, often those with long and complex histories, require the addition of administrative deciders for limited purposes. Always, however, the involved staff, either by itself or with other individuals or committees, must decide on the facts before the process can proceed.

The medical data interpreted by the medical providers' training, skill, and judgment establish the basis for discussions of prognoses; prognoses form the basis for identifying options for care; and the specific options form the basis for mediating various approaches to the appropriate plan of care for the patient.

### Preparing for the Mediation

*Identifying the decision-maker(s) and determining whether the patient is decisionally capable.*   The issue of patient capacity—the patient's ability to consent to or refuse care—is critical. In cases where the patient lacks such capacity, the existence or absence of an advance directive, the appropriate surrogate, and the approved state legal process must all be identified.

Every mediator must have a clear and firm notion of how to approach the issue of decisional capacity, including how to raise the issue and how to evaluate the patient's "decision-specific capacity." If the mediator has any doubt about the patient's capacity, a psychiatric consultation may be in order. In most circumstances, however, the nurses who care for the patient will have the best sense of the patient's capacity and when the patient will be more or less lucid. Whereas "capacity" is a clinical judgment, "competence" is a societal presumption that can be rebutted in a court proceeding. Decision-specific capacity is the capacity to make certain decisions, given their risks and complexity, and not others. As the levels of complexity and risk rise, the level of decisional capacity necessary to address the issues rises commensurately. Thus, a patient may be capable of appointing a proxy (a process requiring a relatively low level of capacity) and not capable of choosing among complex medical options. Note, however, that this sliding-scale notion of capacity, while reflecting reality, also, because of its complexity, invites paternalism; if the physician says making a decision requires a higher level of skill than the patient possesses, the patient, and his or her choice, may be disqualified. To further complicate this assessment, a patient's incapacity may be temporary and the mediator will need to balance the urgency of care with the ideal of patient autonomy.

If the patient is capable, the patient has the legal right to decide about his or her own care and in doing so to make wise or foolish decisions. The mediator should be aware, however, that among the reasons for patient refusals of recommended care interventions is misunderstanding about the nature and cause of the condition and about the purpose of the intervention. Lack of trust in the physician may also be the basis for the patient's refusal.

Although capable adult patients have the right to choose whether to consent to or refuse care, many patients cede this authority to others in the family. The fact that patients possess rights does not necessarily mean that they will choose to exercise them alone without the consultation, support, and participation of family members.

The mediator should be aware that in many cases identifying the family as the "decider" and helping the family to process the decision may constitute the guts of the mediation. Sometimes the family's power will be demonstrated by a health care power of attorney or proxy. Most often, however, the state law on surrogate choice will turn to the family when the patient is no longer capable. If it is the family who gets to decide, then any unresolved ambiguities will largely be resolved by them.

***Determining who should be at the table.***   Once the mediator has met with the treatment team to establish the medical facts, assessed the time constraints, identified the decision makers, and met with the patient and the patient's family, or both, the mediator must determine who should participate in the mediation. During the assessment process the mediator will have determined who are the parties—the ones with the disagreement. The mediator will also know who has information critical to understanding the situation and who has authority to make decisions.

The mediator also must consider whether all members of the treatment team should attend the formal mediation or whether only some members of the team should participate. This decision will turn on such factors as team members' schedules, relationships with the patient and family, who can best present medical facts and treatment options, the desire to avoid overwhelming the patient or family with "white coats," who has power, and who is most emotional or most invested in the case.

Given the complex nature of bioethics mediation and the number of involved parties in a hospital setting, one obligation of the mediator is to see at the outset that all of the relevant parties are included.

*Determining what additional supports are necessary.*    The mediator also should determine whether the patient or the family requires additional supports in preparation for forging an agreement about a care plan. In some cases, the patient or family might need discussions with a social worker or assistance from a psychiatrist consultation-liaison service for anticipatory bereavement counseling. Sometimes clergy or the bioethics committee can be helpful. Case consultation has traditionally been considered one of the functions of a bioethics committee, and it may be that in the context of mediation, the committee could make some of its members available to meet with patients and families to support them through the process of deciding.

*Discussing the decision-making process with a decisionally capable patient.*    If the patient is capable of making medical decisions, it is important to discuss whether there are members of the family or close friends whom the patient would like to have involved in the process of discussion and decision making and what limits, if any, there are from the patient's point of view in discussing the diagnosis and prognosis with these individuals.

The doctrine of informed consent is designed to ensure that a decisionally capable patient who has the legal right to decide about care has the opportunity to consider the relevant information—diagnosis, prognosis, risks, and benefits of alternative treatments—before choosing a medical path. The patient must be capable of making medical decisions and be able to apply personal values to the decision at hand and to communicate the results of this emotional and intellectual process. While the literature discusses these issues under the notion of "informed consent," the more useful term may be "advised consent," which makes it clear that the physician is not the mere conveyor of information but a participant in the decision process whose job it is to advise and guide the patient.

So too, while the doctrine of informed consent contemplates and supports the patient's choosing and provides the legal support for the patient's choice, it does not sentence the patient to deciding alone if he or she chooses to involve others. Some patients are isolated, have no family, and have outlived friends. For these the decision of what treatment to accept or reject is a difficult and solitary exercise. Many patients, however, have devoted family and friends who are available and would like to be involved in considering the options for care. Which of these persons should be invited into the process of discussion and decision is a choice for the patient to make. Members of the care team can help by raising these issues and offering the patient various options for participants in the discussions.

*Identifying family members and friends who may seek to participate in decisions.* Some families form a coherent whole and it is clear what the relationships are and how the emotional architecture of the family has been constructed. In other families the relationships are uncertain and contested. If, for example, there is a patient with a legal spouse from whom she is separated and another man who claims to be the common-law husband and if discord and disagreement exists between these two about what the patient, who is now moribund, would have wanted, the right of one of these two men to speak for the patient must be determined before the conversation about a care plan may go forward. If there is disagreement among adult children about the preferences or prior stated wishes of a now-incapacitated patient, these issues must be sorted out before a plan for deciding can be established. They can, themselves, be matters to be separately mediated or the subjects for caucuses.

Intrafamilial conflict is one of the most toxic and disorganizing elements of a dispute. Sometimes it can be mediated; sometimes it is intractable. The mediator may need to request a decision from legal counsel regarding which member of the family is the legal decision maker.

*Arranging a location for the mediation.*   Mediators often have limited choices about room setup or seating arrangements and must settle for a temporarily empty patient room (see Chapter 8). Nonetheless, it is useful to be aware that the location of a mediation can have an impact on the process. For example, removing participants from their normal workplace to a neutral setting where they are unlikely to be interrupted can aid in focusing on the problem. Going to a different location can indicate that the mediation process is a new way of addressing the problem. But in some cases it can be helpful to conduct the mediation in a familiar setting where the participants are more likely to feel comfortable. Intensive care mediations must almost always be conducted on site since staff cannot leave patients and electronic monitors.

To the extent, however, that the mediator has a choice about location and set-up, he or she also needs to decide whether to meet around a table, how to arrange seating, and whether to provide materials such as an easel, calculators, or paper and pens.

The mediator may have little choice about the shape and size of the table. A round table is ideal but not usually available. The size of the table makes a statement about formality. A large table may create undesirable distance between the parties or the parties and the mediator but it may also establish a zone of safety by separating feuding parties.

Seating arrangements also are significant, especially in bioethics disputes, which involve several parties. The mediator must decide whether he or she wants to break up unproductive alliances, increase the comfort level of participants by seating them with supporters, or encourage new channels of communication by seating people next to those with whom they might have differences. Mediators also should think about who they want talking to whom informally during breaks and try to arrange seating to support those choices.

While mediators may influence communication dynamics by arranging seating, they may, instead, choose to allow participants to determine seating on their own. Watching where parties sit will often give the mediator information about connections and aversions and, in a multisession mediation, watching for changing seating patterns can give the mediator important clues about shifts in positions and changing alliances.

Finally, in the bioethics setting, the mediator should be sensitive to the needs of the patient or patient's family when arranging seating. It may be helpful to seat them next to those members of the treatment team with whom they have the best rapport.

## Stage 2: Beginning the Mediation

Once the mediator has completed the preliminary steps of assessing the situation and preparing for the mediation, he or she moves to Stage 2. In this stage, the mediator usually convenes a meeting of all participants—which mediators refer to as a joint session—and begins to work intensively with both the staff and the patient and family. In a variation of the caucus procedure, the mediator is likely to have already worked, initially, with both groups separately as a way of lowering the intimidation factor for the patient and family and dealing with differences among members of the treatment team.[5] At this stage the expertise of the mediator in managing the mediation process and integrating bioethical principles and legal rules becomes central.

### Introductions

Most mediators begin the mediation session by inviting the participants to introduce themselves to the mediator and to the other parties. Taking time for introductions, or reintroductions, provides a safe and comfortable initial opportunity for all participants to speak and demonstrates the way the mediator will slow down the conversation and check assumptions throughout the mediation session.

The participants can simply identify themselves by name and their role in the dispute and state how they would like to be addressed, or, on a more sophisticated level, they can tell the other participants what they would like them to know about who they are; this introduction can range from facts about their lives to statements about their values, feelings, and goals.

In many bioethics mediations the key player, the patient, is not present. But regardless of whether the mediation involves just the medical team or the team and the family, the mediator should provide an opportunity for the absent patient to be introduced. Too often in the hospital setting the full sense of who the patient is gets lost (see box, p. 61). Making sure the absent patient is "introduced" has several values:

- It reminds everyone of why they are there and that they have a common interest in the well-being of the patient.
- It assures family members of the medical team's concern.
- It may provide important information about what this patient would want.
- It may help the family members clarify their feelings and goals and separate their own emotional reactions from decisions about what the patient would want.

---

5. For a discussion of the caucus procedure, see "Holding Caucuses" in Chapter 5 under "Generating Movement."

- It humanizes the decision-making process.
- It may bring out the fact that there is an advance directive.

### The Mediator's Opening Statement

In the opening statement, the mediator explains the process, sets the tone for the discussion, and begins to build trust.[6] Throughout the process the mediator works to empower parties to reach agreement (or to make an informed choice to pursue non-agreement alternatives); help parties clarify their own goals and priorities; achieve understanding among the parties; and find a fair and wise solution that is stable and durable. In order to achieve these goals the mediator must gain the trust of the parties; demonstrate impartiality, credibility, and authority; and create a safe, comfortable environment. The tone of the mediator's opening statement and the clarity of his or her explanation of the process, participant roles and responsibilities, and ground rules[7] set the stage for productive problem solving (for examples of opening statements, see Chapters 13 and 14).

The bioethics mediator's opening statement differs somewhat from the standard opening statement in classical mediation because the bioethicist should let the participants know that he or she is an employee of the hospital and may offer opinions on ethical and legal issues. Also, the opening statement should note that the "rules" about confidentiality in bioethics mediation differ from those in classical mediation (see p. 26). It should usually cover the following topics.

- *The mediator's role.* The mediator is impartial and will not take sides or advocate for a particular outcome. The mediator is not a judge and will not say who is right and who is wrong, or tell the parties what to do. The mediator will try to understand each participant's concerns and goals and help the participants understand each other's views and plan for the future.

  So, for example, it would be appropriate to begin a bioethics mediation by introducing oneself as "the mediator," saying something like, "I am often called in difficult cases where there are differences of opinion to see whether there is some common ground all can live with. I want to help you figure out what the physicians and nurses think is happening with your mother, what treatment options are available, and what they think should happen in terms of care plan-

---

6. For more on building trust, see Lewicki and Wiethoff 2000.
7. Some mediators prefer the term "guidelines," feeling that "ground rules" sounds too directive.

---

### *"Yes, She Does Seem to Have Been Someone . . ."*

The novel *Moon Tiger*, by Penelope Lively,* begins with the elderly narrator in the hospital and reports the following conversation about her between a nurse and doctor:

> "Was she someone?" enquires the nurse. Her shoes squeak on the shiny floor; the doctor's shoes crunch. "I mean, the things she comes out with. . . ." And the doctor glances at his notes and says that yes, she does seem to have been someone, evidently she's written books and newspaper articles and . . . um . . . been in the Middle East at one time . . . typhoid, malaria . . . unmarried (one miscarriage, one child he sees but does not say) . . . yes, the records do suggest she was someone, probably.

*(New York: Grove, 1987), 1–2.

---

ning. We will then all see together whether any of their suggestions seem right for that person your mother was and is."

- *The process.* The mediator will begin by asking a member of the treatment team to present the medical facts and inviting other team members to add information. Next the mediator will invite the participants to explain their concerns and views of the situation. Then the mediator will ask clarifying questions, help participants to come up with options, evaluate the options, and decide on solutions that will work for all participants.

  Families need to know that the process is ongoing (that they will continue to be consulted) and that whatever is decided in this meeting can be changed in the future if the medical facts change. The process can be used to have an open discussion with all interested parties about various options or to clear up conflicts or ambiguities.

- *Goals.* Most family members and patients and many caregivers have never previously participated in this sort of process. It is important that the mediator help them understand that the purpose of this mediation is to arrive at a treatment plan that can be approved by all, that meets the medical needs and value preferences of the patient, and that satisfies the legal responsibilities of the institution.

- *Disclosure.* The mediator should indicate what information he or she has received prior to the mediation and also reveal any prior contact with any of the participants. The family should be informed if applicable that the mediator has already met with staff for the purpose of helping them discuss the diagnosis and prognosis.

- *Ground rules.* Most mediators ask the parties to listen to each other respectfully and without interruption, while assuring them that each will have a turn to speak. It can be helpful to acknowledge the fact that the parties may have strong feelings or be angry.

- *Confidentiality.* The mediator should inform the participants about confidentiality and its limitations in the hospital setting. In classical mediation parties are assured that what is said in mediation will not be shared with anyone outside the process (or outside the program sponsoring the mediation). In the hospital setting the welfare of the patient depends on information being shared among all those involved in treatment. Therefore blanket promises of confidentiality are inappropriate. However, depending on state law, the mediator may be able to assure the participants that anything that is said in the mediation cannot be used should there be litigation.

- *Final points.* The mediator may want to give an explanation (brief at this point) of what will happen at end of the process: if the parties reach agreement on a treatment plan, it will be entered in the patient's chart; if there is no agreement, alternative processes for making a decision will be explained.

- *Questions.* The mediator's opening statement should end with an invitation to the parties to ask questions about the process.

Once the mediation begins, the mediator should be alert to indications that the patient, family members, or members of the health care team are uncertain about how the process works and offer explanations of the mediation goals and procedures throughout the process.

## Stage 3: Eliciting the Medical Facts

Once the mediator has explained the process, he or she begins the discussion by asking one of the doctors—usually the intern in an academic setting or, in other settings, the physician with the most contact with the case—to describe the case and the patient's history. The mediator may then ask the senior doctor to relay whatever consensus exists on the medical facts (reached at the initial meeting of the mediator and the team), emphasizing the prognosis. (If staff members disagree about the medical facts, the mediator should have the members of the treatment team explain these differences.) Once the medical facts have been stated clearly and completely, the bioethics mediator moves on, and like the classical mediator, gives each participant the opportunity to speak about his or her concerns and helps the parties identify interests, discuss options and principles, evaluate the options, explore preferences, and make decisions about the future. In classical mediation one of the functions of the parties' opening statements is to allow them an opportunity to express strong emotions in a safe and controlled setting. But the mediator must be aware that allowing this opening to become an opportunity for uncontrolled venting can be counterproductive and actually increase anger rather than provide for release of strong feelings (see Allred 2000). At Montefiore Medical Center, the mediators have found it better always to begin mediation sessions with a presentation of the medical facts because allowing family members to let off steam first alienates staff and tends to lock the family members into uninformed positions.

The notion of medical uncertainty is central to all medical decision making and to discussions of prognosis. Nonproviders, however, are unaccustomed to the concept, and little is done to acquaint them with the central place of uncertainty in the practice of medicine. Many providers present the options for care as if each one were as clear and unambiguous as the route of a major interstate highway on a road map. One of the mediator's most important tasks is to help patients and families understand the uncertainty that surrounds diagnosis and treatment. This understanding is a precondition to considering options about care and a critical basis for accepting the outcome, especially if it is the death of the patient.

All bioethics consultants, no matter what their preferred process, agree that "good ethics begins with good facts." Medical facts, in general, are difficult to establish. The very concept of "differential diagnosis" implies multiple possible explanations for the etiology of certain conditions. Often there is disagreement about the origin of a medical condition, the present meaning, and the likely prognosis. So, for example, the patient's kidney function may not be optimal but may be either improving or worsening. It may be that a new medication has caused the problem and that when the medication has been discontinued, the ability of the kidney to function more or less normally will return. Or it may be that the kidney itself is damaged, or that its lack of function reflects problems with other organ systems. The reason for kidney failure will determine how the failure relates to the patient's present condition and likely prognosis. The complexity of this process means that "determining the facts" may involve a lengthy and uncertain chain of discussions. In the course of these discussions, the understanding of the medical facts is refined.

Some "medical facts," such as the patient's history of compliance or noncompliance with prior care plans, are even more difficult to establish. Consider, for example, the following two sets of facts:

1. A patient with infectious multi-drug-resistant tuberculosis refused to remain in his room in the hospital, wandered into the hall, and was finally restrained to prevent him from endangering the other patients and staff.
2. A patient with infectious multi-drug-resistant tuberculosis was put in a negative-pressure room to ensure maximum protection for the other patients and staff. The room was cold, and the patient was denied extra blankets. He was provided with neither a radio nor a television and he had nothing to read. There was no telephone in his room and he ventured into the hall periodically to use the telephone there.

In the first statement of the facts, the staff would be entirely within its rights to restrain a dangerous patient to prevent harm to others. In the second, the right answer is less certain. The staff might still need to act to protect others, but it would also need to meet the needs of the patient and satisfy the demands of a just solution.

The bioethics mediator brings a unique epistemological filter to resolving disputes. Mediators, in general, must be focused on interpreting facts as proposed by the parties. Shame, denial, self-interest, embarrassment, and fantastical thinking often prevent the participants in mediation from making clear presentations. A successful mediator must process the information provided and help the parties evaluate their own positions realistically against a normative notion of reality. This interpretation of facts is by no means unique to bioethical mediation. What bioethics mediation adds is the notion that the "facts" themselves are evolving constantly as the process unfolds. Most bioethics mediations involve patients whose medical condition is uncertain or unstable. What seems to be the reality about diagnosis and prognosis on one day may be totally different on the next. This shifting basis for discussion provides one of the more frustrating contexts for the bioethics mediation process.

During this fact-eliciting stage, the mediator must always keep in mind that "the doctor speaks doctor and the nurse speaks nurse and nobody speaks patient" (Marcus 1992). Medical care providers commonly think in terms of organ function, although some frame the issue in more holistic terms. But it is relatively alien to medical culture to disaggregate the care discussion in terms of the parties and their coinciding or conflicting goals and perspectives. The mediator must bridge the linguistic, cultural, ethnic, and professional gulf that often separates patients and families from providers. It is the task of the mediator to speak to the patient and the family in language they can fathom, using concepts they can understand. The mediator must take into account that different cultures and different ethnic groups have very different patterns of communication.[8] In speaking with an Asian family, for example, the required conventions of discourse may be very different from those used in discussing difficult issues with an African American or an Italian American family. And, of course, all families have their own habits of communication, as well as a private culture known only to them. The mediator must be sensitive to all of these issues in helping the family to understand the medical facts and options and to articulate their values, preferences, and wishes.

In this cacophony of voices, all of the parties are likely to express the idea that they are "speaking for the patient." But it is important to separate the song lines in this chorus of voices to see whether the patient is capable of sufficiently strong self-expression or whether some amplification of his or her voice is required. The physician who advocates for the patient might really be advocating for his own solution. The nurse might actually be in pursuit of administrative order. The family member may be in pursuit of the same dysfunctional or scapegoating arrangements that have long been in place. One might think that a patient's advance directive would be just the vehicle for bringing the voice of the patient to the table. But experience shows otherwise. Living wills, which seem as though they would be best suited to helping the parties reach a decision in any specific case, are often close to, but not actually on, the decision target, leaving considerable discretion to the physician who must decide whether the "trigger" of the document has been satisfied. Although living wills are now less likely than in the past to offer such incomprehensible phrases as "No heroic measures," they are likely to say something equally difficult to interpret, given the changing nature of "medical facts," such as, "If I am unable to make decisions and my doctors say that I will not recover."

A proxy appointment is generally but not always more effective in bringing the voice of the patient to the table. Even if one member of the family is appointed as the proxy, family dynamics, as much as the voice of the patient, are likely to determine what characteristics of the patient and what statements of the patient will be shared with the care team. Dysfunctional families tend not to improve in stressful situations where life and death decisions must be confronted. What Mama said is likely to be less important than the consensus that the family can reach about what she might have wanted in the context of what outcome they can live with. (For a

---

8. For a dramatic and beautifully written story of cross-cultural miscommunication in a medical setting see Fadiman 1998. See also Chew 2001; Kimmel 2000.

robust and engaging review of the conflicted role of the proxy and the obligations that care providers have to these greatly burdened emissaries, see Symposium 1999.)

## Stage 4: Gathering Information

Once the mediator has given the opening statement and elicited the medical facts, he or she invites each party to speak. Then the mediator summarizes what has been said, checks to be sure that the summary is accurate, and begins to ask questions in order to explore and clarify underlying interests.

### *Inviting Statements by Participants*

A good strategy in this stage is to let each party speak without interruption (even by the mediator), until each has explained his or her view of the situation and concerns. As the parties speak, the mediator listens for issues, interests, and feelings, keeping in mind that a person's interpretation of information is based on individual values, life experience, and perception. Using the techniques and tools discussed in the following chapters, the mediator helps the parties create a mutually acceptable definition of the problem and of the issues and interests that should be discussed. Only when the parties agree on what the problem is can they begin to work toward a creative solution.

### *Identifying Issues, Interests, and Feelings*

The mediator must keep in mind, while listening to the parties, that people in conflict are likely to present their stories in the form of threats and generalities (Shaw 2000), taking positions about how they want the problem solved and then digging in and defending those positions. Often the positions that parties take initially do not address all of the issues and fall far short of satisfying their interests. Thus, when all the parties have spoken, the mediator provides an initial summary of the information, reframing in terms of the issues, interests, and feelings rather than just repeating positions. The mediator's task is to probe deep enough to identify the underlying interests of the parties and the issues that must be resolved in order to satisfy those interests.

   How the issues are "framed" reflects a number of problematic assumptions too rarely confronted in bioethical discussions. First, it assumes that all is known that needs to be known when the hint of a dispute first appears. And second, it assumes that the rules and principles that apply will inexorably lead to a single conclusion.

---

### *Issues and Interests*

- *Issues* are the concrete things—behavior, allocation of resources, or future action—that must be dealt with in order to solve the problem.
- *Interests* are the concerns or needs of the parties that are threatened by failure to resolve the issues and that must be satisfied if the solution is to be workable (see box, p. 68). Issues tend to be substantive, psychological, or procedural. Substantive interests might involve goods, time, money, or other resources. Psychological interests typically involve respect, safety, and face-saving—how parties feel about what they experienced. Procedural interests focus on being heard and feeling a decision was made fairly (Menkel-Meadow 2001).

---

But the medical facts, especially the prognosis, and an accurate medical and psychosocial history are often difficult to uncover. Thus, for example, a patient who refuses care may be responding to his relative penury or his lack of trust in the provider or his misunderstanding of the risks and benefits of the proposed intervention. Only knowledge of the context and investigation of the actual circumstances can produce a fair and just result in an individual case.

Once the mediator has identified the issues and interests and summarized them to be sure that nothing has been omitted, he or she then sets the agenda for the discussion by proposing which issues to discuss and in what order. In the case of a complaint about noise from the apartment upstairs, for example, that escalated into a screaming match the next morning in front of the neighbors, the issues are the sounds coming from the upstairs apartment and the ways the neighbors communicate. The interests of the downstairs neighbor may be in getting enough sleep, having quiet when her children are doing their homework, and being treated with respect by her neighbor. The upstairs neighbor's interests might include being able to live as she chooses when in her apartment, having her children able to play without fear of the downstairs neighbor, and also being treated with respect. In bioethics cases issues are likely to include the number and intensity of interventions and the interests of the family in ensuring the comfort of the patient.

How does the mediator decide what to attend to and what to ignore? The mediator is constantly trying to clarify what is important to the participants. People do not always list issues in order of importance; in fact, they often bury the most important information because it is sensitive, they fear it will not be credited, or

---

### *Identifying Interests*

A 78-year-old patient with undetermined and possibly fluctuating capacity is refusing cardiac bypass surgery that her surgeon states is immediately needed to avoid death. She does not want to die but states that she does not feel bad, has things to do at home, and will not agree to surgery now. "Maybe later," she says, "when I am sicker, but not now."

   The issue is whether this woman has the mental capacity to make this choice that will certainly put her life at risk. The parties and their interests include

- the patient, who if capacitated has an interest in self-determination and autonomy, and if decisionally incapable has an interest in being protected from her own inadequate cognition and consideration;
- the patient's children, who have an interest in keeping their elderly mother alive;
- the cardiac surgeon, who has an interest in promoting the best interest of the patient; and
- the consulting liaison psychiatrist, who has an interest in making the correct diagnosis of the patient's capacity so that if the patient is incapacitated the psychiatrist may help to determine and effectuate a plan in her best interest.

---

they may not realize its significance. So if they list four issues that are important to them, the fourth may be the issue to which they give highest priority. The mediator should be aware of this possibility when determining how best to assist the parties. This knowledge may also help the mediator assess what is useful information. One way to determine which issues are really important to the parties is to attempt to assign priorities when setting the agenda for discussion. If the mediator puts an issue at the end of the list or even leaves out an issue, a party for whom the issue is important will usually point out the omission; the mediator can quickly apologize and re-introduce the issue or move it up on the agenda. If the party allows the mediator to leave out the issue, the likelihood is that the issue was being used as a negotiating strategy and is not one of the real interests of the party. Sometimes the mediator must be alert to issues not seen as immediately relevant to the case. For example, cost concerns, allocation, and rationing issues are often present in our health care system but rarely identified clearly in decisions about a particular patient. If these issues are triggered by the case, as they often are, the mediator must be prepared to identify them and to discuss them. Also, as new technologies develop (air fluidized beds, for example, puffed by random air currents that relieve pressure and prevent skin breakdown and bed sores), administrators with limited budgets who have experienced soaring costs from newly introduced technologies in the past are cautious about permitting general unreviewed use of these technologies. Thus, even without widespread health care reform, expensive resources are being administratively recategorized as scarce for the purposes of cost-control.

As the mediation process evolves and mediators listen for and play back to the parties what they have heard, expressing their understanding of the interests and proposed resolutions, participants may acquire information or insights that allow them to modify their positions and their views about what is necessary to resolve the problem.

Many parties in a mediation are experiencing strong feelings. In bioethics disputes the patient and family are wrestling with what are often life-and-death decisions. Members of the medical team, while perhaps less willing to acknowledge it, also often have strong feelings. Most medical professionals take pride in their ability to communicate with patients, families, and co-workers. Research suggests, however, that physicians' poor communication skills are the source of most medical malpractice litigation (Levinson et al. 1997; Hickson et al. 1992). When those communications break down and disagreements develop, the dispute can move beyond the objective facts about what should happen and trigger identity issues for all participants (Stone, Patton, and Heen 1999). Mediators need to help the participants deal with their emotions. One of the most useful ways to do so is simply to acknowledge the feelings being expressed by saying, for example, "Dr. Post, it sounds like you are very concerned about patient Benson and it is hard to find his family so angry and mistrustful," or, "Mr. Adjubi, I can hear how horrible it is for you to be told how sick your daughter is." When participants remain angry or unproductively emotional even after feelings have been acknowledged, the mediator needs to check his or her working hypothesis (see below, "Developing a 'Working Hypothesis'") to see whether it needs to be revised and to consider asking directly what would help. Ultimately, the mediator may have to redirect the participants' attention from emotive behavior if it is not moving them toward their goals.

### *Educating the Staff, Patient, and Family about the Relevant Legal and Ethical Principles*

It is sometimes appropriate for the mediator to spend time during the opening explanation of the process identifying the legal and ethical principles that are relevant to a resolution of the case and begin discussing with the staff and the patient or family how a balance of competing interests might be achieved. The mediator can begin by characterizing the goals of the meeting—"We have to figure out with you what's best for [the patient]"—and then go on to describe what is known, and what bioethical and legal boundaries must be recognized. For example, the intervention may have been precipitated by a situation in which the patient cannot practically (given reimbursement constraints) remain in the hospital for much longer, and the purpose of the intervention is to choose a new location for the patient. But an in-depth discussion of those principles and how they apply to the case being mediated is unlikely to be productive until after the medical facts have been presented and each participant has had the opportunity to speak about his or her concerns.

One way of proceeding from a particular case to the general teaching mandate is to identify key discussions in the legal and ethical literature, explain their arguments, and, if possible, follow up the discussion by distributing a copy of the relevant article or legal opinion. Medical discussions are generally peppered with articulated footnotes to recent and relevant articles in the literature. The closer this mediative discussion conforms to that model, the more comfortable the staff will be.[9]

### Developing a "Working Hypothesis"

Early in the process of information gathering, the mediator will inevitably begin to formulate a working hypothesis, a set of tentative suppositions about the interests of the parties, the issues that need to be discussed, and the likely sources of the dispute. In formulating a hypothesis, the mediator, alert to how the parties interact, draws on all of the information that emerged in the preparation stage, including what the parties have said and what he or she has heard behind their words, as well as knowledge of the institution and life experience. The formulation of a working hypothesis is not a one-time event. The hypothesis continues to evolve, helping the mediator to organize first forays into a case and guiding later interventions.

When and how should that hypothesis be changed, shaped, enriched, supported, strengthened, or overturned during the process? How should it be affected by family dynamics and by the personalities of the care providers? Consider the following case.

A 37-year-old patient with AIDS who has lapsed into unconsciousness is diagnosed with cancer. The oncologist wants to treat the cancer aggressively and the

---

9. One problem is that the style of the long and discursive articles that form the corpus of the medical ethics literature and law cases is quite distinct from the style of most medical writing. There are, however, an increasing number of articles in standard peer review medical journals on bioethics topics that are generally well received by medical staff.

internist, who has been following the patient during his illness, is very suspicious of this strategy. The family is opposed to treatment.

The working hypothesis for the mediator was, "Another case of an overly optimistic and aggressive oncologist who sees only the illness and not the totality of the patient's care needs." (It is important to note that this hypothesis reflects the mediator's bias, prejudice, and past experience, rather than the facts of the case.) As the case evolved, however, it became clear that the parents were afraid that their son's pain and suffering would be increased with treatment. Once they were assured that he would be treated for pain, they began to characterize him as a fighter who wanted every chance, however small, so that he might see his own daughter grow up a bit more. The internist, who was jealous of her turf, began to see the possible benefit of the treatment for the malignancy and acceded to a plan that would, at the very least, begin treatment and evaluate its effect at regular intervals. The working hypothesis changed as the dynamic unfolded and the evidence accumulated. It changed too as the family revealed more about the patient and his feelings and values. As this hypothesis changed, the options that the mediator helped the participants identify continued to evolve to meet the needs of the conversation. The resolution, time-bound and tentative, was to begin treatment and monitor the progress of the patient very carefully to ensure that treatment did not continue longer than was medically justified and that the pain and discomfort of the patient were addressed. (See Chapter 14.)

Every mediator develops a working hypothesis about what is occurring in every session. Without a working hypothesis, it would be difficult for the mediator to know which of many lines of questioning to pursue. It is critical, however, that these provisional theories, even if they are well-grounded, not be permitted to obscure the actual facts and dynamics of the case. Mediators are always testing hypotheses and must be capable of correcting them as necessary during the mediation as new information is provided. They must be careful not to allow their working hypothesis to drive premature solutions and to reevaluate the situation continually as facts "change" and evolve.

Active listening is an important way of checking on the accuracy of the working hypothesis. The mediators listen closely to what the parties are saying, summarizing to test shared understanding and to ensure that other participants have heard, and trying to move the mediation in the direction indicated by the parties. It is important for mediators to determine, continually, what the parties' goals and priorities are and to respond accordingly as they try to help them focus on the future.

Mediators should be alert to signs that their hypotheses are incorrect. When parties are resistant or hostile to mediator interventions, continually repeat themselves,[10] or reject options that seem reasonable or workable, it is likely that the mediator has missed a critical point and should revise the hypothesis.

## Stage 5: Problem Solving

Once the mediator has identified and summarized the issues and underlying interests, he or she moves into the problem-solving stage of mediation. During this stage the mediator helps the patient and family understand the medical facts, assimilate the possible consequences, measure the range of outcomes against shared values, and evaluate and choose options in response to medical questions. Only after this educating process will the patient, or more likely the family, understand the possible tradeoffs in the medical decision-making process. The mediator asks questions to help the parties gain clarity about their interests and goals. One important role of the mediator at this stage is sorting out which interests the parties have in common, which are complementary, and which are in conflict (Menkel-Meadow 2001). As the mediator leads the parties through a discussion of the issues and their interests, options for resolving their differences begin to emerge. (See Chapter 5 for a full discussion of the techniques that are most useful at this stage of the mediation.)

### Managing Discussion

During the mediation process, the mediator sets the agenda by proposing issues for discussion. He or she guides the parties in an exploration of options, encouraging brainstorming so that a range of solutions is considered. Then the mediator works with the parties as they evaluate the options and helps them think about whether and how well various options meet their interests. The mediator also helps parties set priorities and make choices about trade-offs.

Often people experience conflict as chaotic and out of control. They may feel overwhelmed and pessimistic, even hopeless, about finding solutions. These normal tendencies are likely to be heightened in the hospital setting, where people may be confronting what is in fact a hopeless medical prognosis. As the mediator guides the parties through the discussion, proposing topics for discussion, he or she

---

10. Though repetition may also be a sign of insufficient active listening.

replaces the chaos with order by maintaining a calm and calming presence and by being patient and optimistic about the likelihood of crafting a shared solution. The mediator also helps by breaking what seems like an insurmountable problem into manageable pieces for discussion. As in earlier stages, the mediator must be alert to the differing needs of the participants, keeping in mind that it is unlikely that the problem solving will proceed in a linear manner and that "feelings are facts" that must be acknowledged throughout the discussion.

### Developing Options

One of the greatest values that the mediator in bioethics or any other setting adds is help in developing and exploring options.[11] Often the first ideas for solving any problem (usually presented as positions) are based on limited or inaccurate information, erroneous assumptions about the meaning and significance of data, or skewed perceptions. As the parties in a mediation exchange information, examine assumptions, and compare perceptions, a range of possible solutions is likely to emerge. Even when options are limited the exchange can help parties fine tune the alternatives to more closely satisfy their interests.

A mediator might ask a family the following questions about the patient who is not able to be involved in discussions:

- What did [the patient] say to you about any of these issues?
- If you have never talked with [the patient] about [the current issue], knowing what you do about him as a person—his likes, his fears, his values, and his commitments—what do you think he would want?
- What do you and your extended family think about the issues?
- How can we help you to address these issues? What more information might we provide that could be helpful? Could any of the staff be useful in facilitating discussion?

### Shaping Solutions

In the problem-solving phase of the mediation, the bioethics mediator should ensure that all possible solutions are identified and discussed. He or she helps the parties understand the advantages and limitations of proposed courses of treat-

---

11. But presenting people with several options can also make it difficult for them to select the value-maximizing solution. See Guthrie 2003.

ment, the implications for the patient and family of the available options, and whether—and, if so, how—the values and goals of all participants—patient, family, and members of the treatment team—can be reconciled.

### Helping Parties Make Choices

In some mediations, participation in a mediator-guided discussion provides the parties with new understandings of the reasons for behaviors that were upsetting, and that exchange of information alone is sufficient to resolve the conflict. In many more cases, once information has been exchanged, understanding enlarged, and options generated and evaluated, the parties will still have differing preferences. In such situations, the mediator facilitates the negotiation about what action should be taken to resolve the matter.

## Stage 6: Resolution

By the time Stage 5 is completed, the discussion will have reached one of three places.

- Agreement has been reached on all issues.
- It is clear that the parties will not be able to reach agreement.
- Another session is needed because of time constraints or because parties need more time to think or get more information.

### Mediator's Role When Agreement Is Reached

Once participants are able to reach an agreement, the mediator still has work to do. He or she should check with the parties to ensure that the terms are realistic, that the agreement does not contain hidden traps that will cause problems in the future, and that it will, in fact, meet party interests. This is called testing the agreement. The mediator also should check on who will be responsible for which actions, timing, and other details. For example, consider the case of a dispute among members of a medical team about whether an elderly patient, Mr. Hadoni, should be discharged, as he wished, to his isolated rural home or to a nursing home as his physician was urging (see Chapter 9 for the complete case story). During the mediation (which Mr. Hadoni did not attend), his nurse, fearing for his safety if he were allowed to go home, accused the physician of placing financial considerations before the patient's well-being. After discussion, the accusations stopped and all members of the treatment team agreed that Mr. Hadoni, who did not want to be sent to the nursing home where his wife had died, was competent, had the right to control his final days, and should be allowed to die at home. At this point the mediator needed to test the agreed-on decision by asking what services Mr. Hadoni would need, how long it would take to get the pieces of a discharge plan in place, and who would make contact with those who would be providing home care. It was tempting to assume, once the general agreement about where Mr. Hadoni would go was reached, that the normal procedures for putting a discharge plan into place could be relied on. It works better, however, if the mediator makes sure that all participants know what their roles will be in implementing the agreement.

The final responsibility of the mediator, then, after acknowledging the efforts made by all participants, is to review the decisions about the treatment plan and the responsibilities of each participant in carrying out the plan and to enter the agreement in the patient's chart. Sometimes it is even prudent to give the non-institutional parties a non-institutional copy of the chart note, although some risk managers may object to this practice.

### Mediator's Role When There Is No Agreement

If it is clear that the parties will not be able to reach agreement, the mediator has several responsibilities. In classical mediation the mediator needs to help the parties consider whether some other dispute resolution process would work for them and think about what their next steps should be (making a final offer, seeking counseling, consulting a lawyer). In the bioethics context, the parties are not the ones who decide what decision-making process will be used to resolve their differences. Therefore the bioethics mediator should be sure each participant understands what will happen next in order to resolve the dispute and who will be making the decisions. There are several configurations for the deciders, but most will include a risk manager, an administrator, and, sometimes, hospital counsel.

The mediator might also thank the participants, acknowledging their efforts and the difficulty of the situation but also validating any progress made during the mediation by noting any increased understanding, exchange of information, or clarification of concerns. Some mediators make themselves the scapegoat, saying, "I'm sorry I have not been able to help you more." If the mediator is comfortable with this approach, it can help the participants by relieving them of responsibility for not reaching agreement. In cases where the need for a decision is not urgent, the mediator can suggest that the parties let the situation percolate for a while so they can consider new information and a new range of options.

### Mediator's Role When Another Session Is Required

At times the parties will have made progress but need to have additional mediation sessions because the issues are too complex to resolve at one sitting; emotions are raw and need time to heal; additional information is needed; the participants need time to process new information; outside advice is needed (from, for example, a family member, counselor, member of the clergy, or lawyer); or the parties may want to try out some tentative agreements, both to test their feasibility and to build trust. It may be especially useful to schedule a follow-up session to evaluate tentative agreements where the mediator or one or both parties have doubts about the viability of a proposal. Building into the mediation process a time to return to the table and revise or abandon a trial solution may avoid having the parties feel that they have failed or that one of them has not followed through on the terms of the agreement.[12]

When another session is agreed upon, the mediator should end the current session by summarizing the discussion, including any provisional agreements and any tasks to be completed before the next session. At the beginning of each subsequent session the mediator should begin with a brief opening statement, reviewing the mediation process and progress to date.

### What Constitutes a Successful Outcome in Bioethics Mediation

In bioethics mediation the process is a part of the product. A successful mediation is one that incorporates all or some of the following characteristics:

- Demonstrates respect for all of the participants
- Assists the participants in understanding each other
- Ensures that no one party dominates the conversation, intimidates the others, or bars appropriate topics from discussion
- Identifies patient rights or values that might have been overlooked in prior segments of the decision-making process
- Translates the language of the medical staff into the language of nonmedical persons, thereby demystifying the discourse
- Categorizes and arrays overlapping concerns
- Maximizes the options that will be considered

---

12. See Chapter 8 for an example, in the context of a bioethics mediation, where a tentative agreement about visiting hours did not work out.

- Allays the anxiety of the patient or family, to the extent possible, and directs attention to the actual medical choices being faced
- Facilitates the ongoing discussion of the options that might be acceptable as solutions and probes to see whether some of these options might be more acceptable if time-limited or approached in a specific sequence
- Helps patient, family, and staff to evaluate these options in terms of relevance to the patient's values and feasibility within the changing medical condition of the patient
- Buys time for interim solutions as the medical facts evolve

These end points are the marks of a successful mediation whether or not an agreement is reached among all of the parties. If there is a governing consensus reached, however, there is one last crucial requirement: that the solution forged comport with the notion of a "principled resolution" (see box, pp. 78–79).

Finally, there is an additional measure of success that, to some degree, stands in contrast to the factors detailed above. A successful mediation may occur when the mediator acknowledges that the situation is not appropriate for mediation and that there are well-accepted legal rules and ethical principles that must be applied.

At that point the consultant role of the bioethics mediator/consultant must become dominant and the outcome that is dictated by rules and principles must be ensured. Bioethics mediators/consultants must be alert to the process. They must always remain neutral and open-minded regarding the outcome. Nonetheless, they are not indifferent to the outcome. They may and should, whenever appropriate, reformulate the options to satisfy the needs and interests of the parties. They must be ever mindful, however, of the rights of the parties and be ready, when appropriate, to act in support of the rights of patient and family.

Once an agreement is reached, the mediator reviews the terms with the parties. Finally, in classical mediation, the mediator checks with the parties to see whether a written agreement is needed and, if so, depending on the setting, drafts either the agreement or a memorandum of agreement and reviews the language with the parties. In bioethics mediation, any agreement is entered by the mediator in the patient's chart.[13] If there is no agreement, the mediator in any setting discusses the next steps to be taken by the parties. In bioethics mediation, he or she documents that discussion in the chart.

---

13. If an outside mediator is used, it will be necessary to have someone else write the chart note.

## Sample Chart Note

### The Case

This case involved a 54-year-old woman with recurrent breast cancer who had put off treatment until the lesion had developed into an open and foul-smelling wound. She had been married less than a year before and she was committed to keeping her "secret"—the fact that she was dying—to herself. Her husband was committed to the same process of secrecy. The consult was called by the surgical resident who was in charge of the patient's care, although it had been determined by the surgical attending that there was no possible surgical intervention in this case. The patient had been admitted to the hospital from the Emergency Department and when it was observed that there was bleeding from the tumor, she was admitted to surgery. At the time of the consultation, the patient was receiving dressing changes, transfusions for blood loss, and radiation, all of which were palliative. Each time the dressings were changed there was extensive bleeding. Diagnostic tests had indicated widespread metastases to the brain, spine, bones, liver, and pancreas. Despite the diagnosis and prognosis, in conversations with the husband, he requested that the tone of talk with the patient be "upbeat." Part of the problem was that this consultation was the Wednesday before Thanksgiving and the patient's primary oncologist was not available. The staff, in general, was feeling undersupported and somewhat depressed at being in the facility at the start of the holiday. Understaffing in surgery made the resident feel particularly beleaguered. The mediator met first with the care team, then with the husband alone, then with the wife-patient alone, and then with the couple together. She then wrote the chart note.

### The Chart Note

This is a patient who is dying and who refuses to accept the diagnosis. Her husband is also either in denial or unable to face the reality [of her death] with his wife.

*Question #1:* Is the patient decisionally capable?

The patient is clearly oriented X3 [to time, person, and place] but in denial about her condition. Some would argue that this sort of pathological denial indicates incapacity. But, in this case, misinterpreted medical statements (like the purpose of radiation is to "shrink" the tumor) fueled unrealistic hopes.

*Suggestion #1:* Get radiology to talk with patient and husband about the purpose of treatment being palliative.

*Question #2:* How can we pierce the denial to help the patient and her husband deal with the reality that approaches?

*(continued on next page)*

Good decisions are based on a level of understanding of the options and a measuring of those options against the values of the patient. In this case the patient does not want to give up. The husband supports this (although a conversation alone with him after the consult indicates that he knows that she is dying).

*Question #3:* How can you help to structure clear decision making in these conditions?

One other factor is critical. Dr. P— and the other surgical residents are a scarce resource and that needs to be protected for other patients in the service. Dr. P— and I agreed that there are three appropriate places to manage the care of the patient: the long-term care facility associated with the hospital, the hospice unit, or the AO [attendings only] service that does not use house staff as providers. The patient and her husband agreed that they will consider all of these options.

I would argue that the decisions presented to the patient and her husband should be confined to medically appropriate options. (I will be in touch with the assistant to the medical director and with the nurse on Palliative Care to alert them to the discussions.) I was in touch with the patient's oncologist, who agreed, even though he is away from the hospital, to accept her in the AO service. Some cases call for boundaries. This is such a case. The choices for the family must be limited by what is appropriate medically. The fact is that no service is eager to assume responsibility for this dying patient on this holiday weekend. Palliative Care will take the lead in trying to find an appropriate service.

*Summary:* This case is a classic example of Bioethics Mediation. There is no real bioethics issue but rather a situation in which patient and family are caught in hard decisions with no real choices. [The following, second, note in the case was added two days later.]

I spoke with Mr. S— this morning, who has stated that we may not speak with his wife about her care and especially about her dying. I explained about the patient's right to choose and he disparaged this issue. I stated that if his wife signed a health care proxy and she agreed that he should assume decision-making authority immediately that we would respect her wishes and hold all future discussions with him.

I have met with the patient and she stated clearly that she wants her husband to make decisions about her care. This idea—called delegated autonomy—is within permissible ethical analyses. This patient does not want to hear about her impending death. We cannot force her to engage with us. Dr. O— [the head of the palliative care team] and I have discussed this case, met together with the patient, and agreed that oblique communication, not direct, is likely to continue. This is a capacitated patient who wants (has chosen) to be passive. She cannot and will not confront her dying. We will need to support her comfort without her clearly accepting or refusing interventions.

### Closing the Session

At the end of any mediation session the mediator should review the decision reached, pausing to get the parties' assent to each element. If the parties have not reached agreement, the mediator should review the issues and interests identified during the mediation and acknowledge progress made during the session. Regardless of the outcome, the mediator should validate the effort and work of the participants and thank them for participating.

### Documenting the Decision in the Patient's Chart

A bioethics consultation or mediation is part of the decision history in any case. In most bioethics mediations, the only written record of the decision made by the group will be the mediator's notes in the patient's chart.[14]

The patient's chart sets and describes the patient's condition at any moment. It is a legal document that cannot be changed or amended after the fact. It is essential that the mediator's notes be clear, legible, complete, and accurate. The notes should describe who participated, what the issues were, and what decision was reached. It may be written on the progress notes in the chart or placed on a special form used by consultants in general.

## Stage 7: Follow-Up

Outside the medical setting, mediators may work with the parties after agreement is reached to help with implementation, for example, serving as the delivery point for an exchange of money or goods or convening continued meetings to adjust and amend agreements to take into account unexpected (or even expected) complications. In the bioethics context, the follow-up stage may involve any of the tasks described below.

### Ensuring That the Agreed-upon Resolution Is Implemented

Ensuring implementation of the resolution may require as little as a note in the medical chart setting forth the decisions reached in the course of the mediation or consultation. It may, however, require some further action by the mediator. Espe-

---

14. Similarly, in classical mediation, although the parties can be assured that their discussions are confidential, any written agreement is not confidential unless the parties include a stipulation to that effect.

cially in a dynamic case, the mediator may need to be in touch with the care team to help it and the patient or family address the changing ethical contours of the case.

### Following-up with Family and Staff to See Whether Support for the Family Is Needed

Some families will be able to reach a decision even if issues among family members and their long-standing unresolved tensions have not abated. It may be that one of the family, on either the "winning" or the "losing" side, may need additional support after the surgery takes place or the ventilator is disconnected. The party making the decision, whether it be a decisionally capable patient or the family of an incapable patient, needs the compassion and support of the staff. Similarly, if the patient is suffering, then that pain and discomfort is an ethical as well as a medical issue. If the patient is no longer suffering, the staff's obligations largely shift to the family.

Physicians and the care provider teams may think that their responsibilities are terminated when the patient is transferred or dies. But studies of family dynamics that focus on the needs of the proxy argue that there is some ongoing obligation to help the family members and the proxy assimilate the facts and feelings about what has occurred. Dubler (1995), for example, has long argued that there are special obligations owed to the formal legally appointed proxy or to the informal surrogate who is empowered within the care setting to make decisions for the patient. Whereas the medical professionals often treat the proxy as a sort of junior colleague when difficult decisions must be faced, the bioethics mediator should keep in mind that the proxy is most often a grieving and disoriented family member who must make decisions in the context of medical uncertainty that will weigh heavily in the future on his or her conscience.

It is often helpful for family members to have spoken with the patient about the patient's wishes, but sometimes these efforts are not possible and sometimes they are unproductive. Receptivity to discussions about possible disability and death varies with culture. And proxies' and patients' abilities to mount these sorts of discussion vary with personality. Whether or not the patient has been able to indicate what would be wanted and whether or not there is a legally appointed proxy, decisions will need to be made about the patient's care. Either these decisions will be made by family members or they will be made by strangers, usually the physician and other members of the medical team. In general, the first is preferable. But the care team must then accept that the process of deciding places grave burdens on those appointed proxies, informal surrogates, and family members who feel responsible for the decisions, especially if the decisions permit or facilitate the death of the patient.

One of the obligations of the mediator that flows from this analysis is the obligation to support the family members in the process of deciding. With this obligation must come an awareness of the fine line between taking over the decision and helping to shoulder the burden of and responsibility for the decision. It is not the role of the mediator or of the care team to usurp the powers of the family to decide. It is the role of the mediator, however, to help the care team shoulder as much of the responsibility for a decision as is feasible. For example, the mediator might help the care team to frame the decision so that the team states, "Your mother is really not a candidate for resuscitation," rather than, "Do you want your mother to be resuscitated?"

### Debriefing Medical Staff on Medical, Ethical, and Policy Issues

When there has been a particularly troubling case, the staff will often have feelings about how the case unfolded and was resolved and how like cases should be handled in the future. They will also need to consider whether there were hospital policies that contributed to the bad outcome and if so how they might be modified.

If there is a sad outcome, the staff may need time and space to express their sorrow and their discomfort, especially with any role that they might have played in the process. Often taking time to sit together and review the conduct of the case, how the events overtook the patient and family, is very helpful. In particularly troubling cases, for example, some involving children, formal rounds is the best forum in which to address sorrows among the staff. At other times, a visit to the nurses' rest area will suffice to gather the team and take a moment to grieve together. If there is an opportunity to review the facts of the case, the medical and ethical choices made, and the resulting outcome, the mere process of review is helpful.

### Highlighting Hospital Policy Issues

If the case has been affected negatively by a hospital policy or procedure, one of the tasks of follow-up is to identify and begin to evaluate the policy. Consider, for example, the sticky issue of the do not intubate order. There are some situations that require a discussion not only of resuscitation but also of intubation, or putting a patient on a ventilator. National standards for resuscitation require that intubating the patient be part of the process. However, there are some patients and families who want resuscitation without intubation and this request presents several problems, including its contradiction of the national standards. Some hospitals have policies that permit patients and families to choose a "partial code," that is, some intervention short of intubation. If a bioethics mediator encounters a situation, for example, where hospital policy precludes this option but it is an option that the family wanted, he or she should raise the issue with the bioethics committee or another forum in the hospital to confirm the policy and discuss whether it needs some emendation.

# 5

## *Techniques for Mediating Bioethics Disputes*

THIS CHAPTER DESCRIBES techniques used by classical mediators,[1] highlighting those that are especially relevant to bioethics mediators.[2] Mediation skills training should be a hands-on experience. Most basic mediation training involves from 24 to 40 hours of experiential, interactive instruction followed, ideally, by an apprenticeship. But all mediators, even the most intuitive and experienced, should keep up with the literature. As the field develops, old assumptions are continually being tested and challenged by researchers, who refine some and disprove others.

In bioethics mediation, as in all mediation, the mediator has to choose what information to reflect back and what is not useful in the context of the goals of the process. Generally, useful information moves the process forward. Each party's explanation and interpretation of the facts and of what he or she hopes to accomplish, as well as his or her understanding of the limits of the process, are important. An effective mediator encourages each party to speak and listen and thus to clarify or even change his or her own position and perhaps to erase any inaccurate perceptions about the position or motives of the other side.

An effective mediator also listens and watches for signals that a party may be receptive to change, intervening with a question or comment for clarification. When mediators are incorrect in their assessments, the parties are usually quick to clarify their positions. It is unlikely that a mediator can force a party to change his or her thinking by inaccurately (from the participant's perspective) summarizing what was heard.

---

1. For a more comprehensive discussion, see Moore 1996; Kressel 2000.

2. There is much debate in the literature about whether mediators should act only as facilitators or also evaluate the merits of parties' claims and whether they should address only the narrow issues presented initially by the parties or probe for broad underlying issues. See Riskin 1996, 2003.

An intriguing and challenging task for any mediator is determining which data are relevant to the mediation process and how much relative attention various factors should be given in the discussions. This evaluation goes on continually, from the initial drawing out of the history of the conflict and the interests of the participants to the later identification and arrangement of options and, finally, to the review of proposed resolutions. The skilled mediator understands the danger, especially in medicine, of prematurely cataloguing "facts" as though they were immutable objects rather than the shifting elements of a dynamic picture that evolves and develops only gradually. The shorthand for this weighing of data is the question, How can we ensure that all relevant information is considered?

This task of sifting and sorting emerging data is made even more complicated for the bioethics mediator by the demands of the clinical setting. Against the backdrop of emotionally charged issues, rapidly changing medical conditions, and numerous concerned parties from diverse backgrounds, the mediator needs a heightened awareness and quick responses to process incoming, often conflicting, information. Moreover, the way in which data are introduced significantly affects how they are perceived. Stories of conflicts are rarely presented as complete narratives. Rather, information comes in bits and pieces, often unrelated, out of order, sometimes inconsistent. When placed together like pieces of a puzzle to create an emerging picture, they may look very different than they did when first offered as fragments. Likewise, the source of the information will influence the importance it is accorded. Indeed, the differing perceptions of events are often precisely what create conflicts. The person requesting the bioethics consultation supplies the introductory version of the disputed situation. This person can naturally be expected to emphasize certain parts of the story, while minimizing or even ignoring others or filtering the information before it even reaches the consultant. When still another group of interested parties is convened, additional information and alternative perspectives are added.

What medical facts, prognostic categories, patient statements, or family memories will be sufficiently compelling to affect the course and conduct of the discussions? The mediator in a bioethics consultation is not a judge. There are no rules of evidence that constrain what can be accorded weight in the process. There are no exclusions from the transcript or from the hearing of a jury; nothing will be struck from the consideration of the parties who must cooperate to forge a consensus. Yet, some statements and some sorts of memories are more relevant than others. The mediator must decide which statements are useful guideposts for the resolution of the conflict and which are barriers to a desirable outcome.

## Summarizing

The mediator is constantly gathering information, testing tentative hypotheses, and summarizing what has been said. The repetitive summary is a key aspect of the mediation process that

- lets the parties know that the mediator has been listening,
- lets the mediator test his or her understanding of what was said,
- helps the parties organize their thoughts,
- helps the parties hear what others are saying,
- shows the parties areas of common interest,
- provides a way to order the discussion, and
- lets the mediator remind parties of progress that has been made.

Mediators can use summarizing simply to be sure that all participants have heard what was said, to focus on particular issues, or to move the discussion forward (for examples, see the transcripts in Chapters 13 and 14). Summarizing may be the most critical mediator skill. It cannot be overused.

In classical mediation, the mediator does not begin to summarize until after all parties have completed their opening statements. Summarizing after only one party has spoken runs the risk of seeming to endorse that speaker's view and often leads to a discussion of or response to it before the other parties have had a chance to be heard. This model is not necessarily appropriate in the bioethics setting, however, because of the importance of establishing the medical facts. To repeat, in bioethics mediations, the mediator usually starts by asking one of the physicians to state the medical facts. Then, typically, the mediator summarizes the medical facts, translating them into lay language if necessary to ensure that the patient or the patient's family understands and checks on whether anything has been omitted or whether there is disagreement (about the data, itself, not about its implications), before moving on to get each participant to speak about his or her concerns and views of the situation.

Participants are likely to have strong feelings and to express those feelings in quite different styles. The mediator should be alert to the feelings of all participants, acknowledge them in the summary, and give permission for their expression but also be aware that unmoderated venting of feelings is likely to be counterproductive (Allred 2000). In the bioethics setting, as in all mediations, if parties remain so emotional that they cannot engage productively in the discussion, the mediator should check to see whether he or she has missed an important issue.

Mediators find it useful to summarize throughout the mediation, especially after an exchange of information, suggestion of possible solution, or expression of emotion. Summarizing is much more than simply playing back the speaker's words. Mediators use summaries to capture in their own words the essence of what has been said, perhaps tying a new statement to earlier statements. They also use summaries to remind parties of their interests, to help bring order to what the parties may be experiencing as a chaotic, unmanageable, out-of-control situation, and to amplify helpful statements while cutting out the biting words. Repeating some of the nondestructive language of the speaker can also be a powerful tool. In addition, summarizing can help mediators who feel stuck by giving them a moment to collect their thoughts and decide what to place next on the agenda for discussion.

The following are useful openings:

- Let me see if I understand what you are saying.
- If I hear you correctly, ——
- So you are saying that ——
- Let me take a minute and try to summarize what you've both been saying.

The mediator can use a summary to point out something the parties have in common.

- So you are both saying that you want to be treated with respect and for you, Ms. A, that means —— and, Mr. B, you would like —— and each of you has some other concerns.
- Ms. A, if I heard you correctly, —— and, Mr. B, you feel ——

Without repeating hostile, hurtful, or attacking words, the mediator can acknowledge the feelings expressed by those words and summarize the information behind them. An effective summary includes issues, interests, and feelings. For example:[3]

*Ms. A:* I brought this complaint because he trapped two of my children in the elevator and threatened them. Now they are terrified of him. He had no right to treat my children like that. If he has problems, he should talk to me. He is crazy—a madman.

---

3. In this chapter we have used nonmedical examples in order to keep the focus on the techniques. Our experience in training is that the facts of medical cases often distract from the focus on skills.

*Mr. B:* The noise from her apartment is unbearable. Her children are like animals. Someone has to tell them how to behave. It is no wonder they don't know how to behave with a bitch like that for a mother. I work hard and have to get up early. I need to get my sleep.

*Mediator's summary:* Let me summarize what I've heard so far. You are both angry and upset [feelings they have in common]. Mr. B, you are concerned about the sounds coming from Ms. A's apartment [issue], and you need it to be quiet enough for you to get your sleep [interest]. And Ms. A, you are concerned about the way Mr. B communicates with your children [issue] and you don't want your children to be afraid of their neighbors [interest]. And you also indicated you would like Mr. A to speak directly with you if he has concerns about your children [proposal]. Is there anything I have missed?

Notice that the mediator ends the summary with a question (a statement can be equally effective) designed to move the discussion forward and avoid creating a pause that the parties could take as an invitation to repeat and embellish what they have already said. The summary allows the mediator to check with the parties to be sure he or she has understood them and, if not, to give them the opportunity to correct any misunderstanding.

In the early stages of a mediation the mediator usually should follow a summary with a clarifying question.

- Mr. B and Ms. A, could you each tell me about your daily schedule, when you and the other people in your apartment get up, what your routines are?
- When you say you want to be treated with respect, what do you mean?

Later in a mediation, after summarizing additional information gained as a result of asking questions to clarify, the mediator may want to ask a further question—based on what the parties have said—that presents an option for solving part or all of the dispute.

> [Summarizing as above.] Given those concerns, do I understand that you both think it would make sense to agree that, Mr. B, when you have concerns about the A children you will tell Ms. A instead of talking to the children?

(If the parties say yes, the mediator would go on to test the agreement by asking how that would work. Would they speak directly? communicate by phone? etc.)

## Questioning

Mediators ask questions for many reasons, including:[4]

- To obtain a broad overview: What brings you here? Tell me more about that. I'm not sure I understand—could you give me more details?
- To obtain information: How much is your rent? Could you describe the layout of your apartment? How old are your children?
- To clarify abstract ideas or generalizations: What do you mean when you say that she never returns your calls? How do you propose to accomplish this? When you say you want to be treated with respect, what do you mean?
- To focus the discussion: How does this relate to the issue of ——?
- To encourage parties to evaluate alternatives: Which of these two options do you consider the best? Do both options work equally well for both of you? What do you see as the advantages and disadvantages of this proposal?
- To learn why a party holds a position: Why do you think ——? How will this solve the problem?
- To introduce a hypothetical idea: Suppose you tried this option, what do you think would happen? What if Mr. C could repair your sofa? Given the nature of the problem, is it possible to ——?
- To generate new options: Are there other ways to solve this problem? If you could write the script, what would it be?
- To encourage participation in the discussion: What do you think about that, Ms. M? How does that idea strike you, Mr. J?

Asking the right questions at the right times and for the right reasons is critical to productive mediation. Choosing the appropriate questioning technique is also important.

- *Open-ended questions* give the speaker the opportunity to say what is important to him or her in whatever form he or she chooses. They also are a way of encouraging the party to speak. (Examples: What brings you here? Tell me your view of the situation. Tell me more about that.)
- *Narrow questions* focus the speaker on a specific topic. (Examples: Tell me about the conversation. What is the layout of your apartment? What is your normal billing procedure?)

---

4. This discussion of the goals of questions is based on Pope 1993.

- *Closed questions* ask for specific information or a yes or no answer. (Examples: What color is your house? What time do your children go to bed? Is that your green car? Do you normally work from nine to five?)

In general, mediators should choose questions carefully, think about their goals in asking the question, and ask only one question at a time. Asking multiple questions gives the person responding a chance to choose which question to answer, and the choice will usually be to answer the easiest and avoid the most difficult questions. However, where the mediator senses that parties are uncertain about what they want to say, using multiple questions invites them to choose from a range of topics, letting them start where they are most comfortable, while still providing some guidance regarding the structure of the discussion.

## Generating Movement

Mediators use several techniques to overcome impasses and keep the discussion moving during the problem-solving stage of the mediation.

### Asking Problem-Solving Questions

Questions that ask the parties to focus on their interests and possible solutions can help move the parties toward resolution.[5] For example, in a dispute between a parent and a teenager about curfew, friends, and other issues, the mediator might ask the mother, "You have said you are concerned about your daughter's safety when you don't know where she is or whom she is with. What could she do to make you less concerned?" Or the mediator could say to the daughter, "You've heard your mother say she is worried about your safety when ———. Do you have any ideas about what you could do to make her less concerned?"

### Reframing

One way that mediators help parties hear each other is to reframe what they have said, dropping biting words (without ignoring the strong feelings that those words represent) and looking beyond statements of position to recognize interests.

*Tenant:* That thieving, no-good scoundrel locked me out of my apartment and then took my stuff. He's going to pay for that.

---

5. See above, p. 90, for a discussion of forms of questions and other purposes of questioning.

*Mediator:* So you are very angry because you believe that your landlord was responsible for your missing property, and you'd like to be compensated. Is that right?

### Raising Issues

It may also be important for the mediator to ask questions about issues that the parties have not addressed explicitly. Parties will often hint at underlying issues or interests as a way of testing whether they can safely be discussed. For example:

- Business partners may have had a falling out and be fighting about how the assets should be divided. The mediator may sense that they are each feeling hurt and betrayed, much like parties to a divorce, and ask them about those feelings.
- An older woman may have said several times, "No one should be spoken to like that. His language was inexcusable," but never specified what was said. The mediator, sensing that the language itself is critical to the dispute, might ask parties whether they would be comfortable telling him or her what was said.
- A young man may have referred at several points to another participant and her family as "those kinds of people." The mediator might ask for clarification, sensing that there are underlying stereotypes that need to be addressed or cultural differences that are having an impact on the dispute.
- In a dispute between neighbors with children who had played together in the past, the mediator might ask about the impact of the dispute or a proposed resolution on the children.

In the bioethics context, the mediator may need to raise the following issues:

- Is the patient suffering? A prime concern for the bioethics mediator is that the patient not suffer unnecessarily. However, in end-of-life situations, if the patient is beyond help or suffering, the balance shifts. At that point, the mediator might concentrate on the needs of the family rather than the needs of the patient.
- Does the family/patient or staff have unrealistic expectations? Should the focus be on palliative treatment? Are one or both of the parties so invested in this case that they are supporting futile treatment?
- Is the family taking up a disproportionate amount of staff time? Is there an issue of the fair allocation of scarce resources?

### Hearing Proposals

Often parties, in the midst of heated and attack-filled statements, make proposals. But the party who made a proposal may not even be aware of having done so and most likely the other party will not have been able to get past the hurtful words to hear it. The mediator should listen for the proposal and then, at the appropriate time—often later in the mediation when the parties are beginning to feel heard and to trust the process—inquire about it.

*Mr. A:* This isn't gonna work. You can't trust that guy for a minute. He's so crooked I'd have to hire someone to watch him the whole time just to make sure he does what he's supposed to.

*Mediator* (later in the process): Are you saying that if Mr. B were supervised in fulfilling his part of the agreement you'd be able to accept these terms?

### Stroking

When mediators talk about stroking they are actually referring to two different techniques: first, acknowledging feelings, and second, recognizing the work of the participants in the mediation. Statements that acknowledge feelings begin with phrases such as, "So you are saying you felt disrespected" or, "You were feeling hurt" or, "It sounds like you were confused and frightened by her reaction."

Statements that give recognition to the parties for their efforts in the mediation process can acknowledge suggestions and offers, the way the parties interact with each other, their willingness to listen or to talk about difficult subjects, the understanding they show of the other's perspective or concerns, or their willingness to make concessions or compromise. A mediator might say, for example, "I know it is difficult to discuss these issues, especially with strangers, and I appreciate your willingness to talk about them" or, "That is a very helpful proposal. I can see you want to work this out" or, "This is a difficult situation. I can see that it is hard for you to be here" or, in response to a concession or change in perspective, "It is helpful that you are willing to consider the problem from his perspective" or, to recognize progress, "It's great you two have agreed on these three points. You're making real progress here."[6]

---

6. Bush and Folger (1994) argue that the goal of mediation should be empowerment and recognition. By empowerment they mean looking for opportunities for parties to make decisions for themselves and by recognition they mean encouraging opportunities to develop an understanding of the other person's perspective. We have found that recognition is often a three-step process. Parties arrive at a mediation feeling uncertain and unworthy. The mediator provides recognition to each party by acknowledging his or her feelings and interests and the impact of the dispute on his or her life. This recognition by the mediator allows the parties to give themselves and their concerns recognition and then perhaps to give recognition to the other party.

### Allowing Silence

Many people have difficulty tolerating silence, but simply sitting quietly, waiting for a response gives people time to think before speaking. Silence can also be a gentle tool for eliciting useful information. Mediators should be aware, however, that some cultures are more comfortable with silence than others.

### Holding Caucuses

Caucuses are private meetings between the mediator and one of the parties or a group of participants with similar interests or goals. Caucuses may be necessary to help the parties articulate their questions, explore the interests underlying their positions, and order their values and preferences. For example, when a party appears intimidated or disempowered, a caucus can provide the emotional, intellectual, and sometimes physical space for quiet contemplation, perhaps allowing him or her to regain emotional composure to better understand the facts, implications, and options. In a caucus, family members can decide how they are going to proceed with the process of decision making. Parties may request that some or all of what is discussed in caucus not be shared with the other party. In bioethics mediation, to repeat, the confidentiality rules are different. However, there are situations in which the mediator will not divulge information told to him or her in private which may be critical to an understanding of the emotional construction but not relevant to the clinical decisions (see Chapter 9).

In some cases, mediators will caucus only once with each party. In other cases, the mediator may use multiple caucuses, sometimes with joint sessions mixed in. Whenever a mediator caucuses with one party, it is important also that he or she meet in private with all others. The possibility of private sessions is best introduced during the mediator's opening statement. There are several reasons to use caucuses:

- To allow expression of strong feelings without increasing the conflict
- To cut off unproductive communication
- To provide an opportunity to discuss the situation without the stress of talking in front of the other participants
- To obtain confidential information
- To clarify issues
- To reality test with one party where doing so in a joint session might make the mediator seem partial to one side
- To avoid reactive devaluation and other psychological phenomena that research has shown can get in the way of finding solutions (Arrow et al. 1995)

- To prevent one or both parties from getting entrenched in early positions
- To explore possible power imbalances
- To address unproductive tactics and coach on how best to use the process
- To allow parties to take risks in generating options and exploring alternatives
- To test a party's bargaining range
- To break a deadlock
- To help a party evaluate a proposal

Mediators should also be aware of potential problems with the use of caucuses. Initially, caucuses may make one or both parties suspicious. Mediators may use caucuses prematurely or too frequently because of their own discomfort with conflict, thereby depriving the parties of the opportunity to work together to address underlying issues and resolve their differences.

### Reality Testing

One of the tasks of a mediator is to help the parties be realistic about their goals and predictions. Reality testing, most often used in caucus, is a technique that encourages parties to abandon extreme positions and think more realistically about possible solutions. One of the most common methods of reality testing is simply to ask what will happen if the problem is not solved. Another, in the face of an extreme demand, is to ask how the person making the proposal thinks the other party will respond.

### Reversing Roles

Mediators can help a party gain insight into possible solutions by asking questions that invite him or her to consider how the other party experienced a particular situation; how he or she would respond if in the other party's shoes; or what he or she thinks the other party will say about an offer. Role reversal can seem closely linked to reality testing but, at its best, goes further and helps parties broaden their perspective on the problem and develop empathy for one another. However, in many disputes parties are too angry to care about or be willing to consider the other's perspective.

### Developing Options

Mediators should remember that the first proposals are rarely the best proposals since they are based on imperfect information. Taking time to explore the parties' interests, gather information, and then develop a range of options often leads to much richer and more nuanced solutions. (Useful studies on brainstorming and generating options include Adams 2001.)

### Normalizing

People in conflict often feel isolated and hopeless because they have never before faced the sort of problem they are facing now and cannot imagine a way out. Simply letting them know that others have found themselves in similar situations and found solutions can be enormously helpful.

### Packaging Proposals

Research has shown that the way people respond to a proposal is influenced by such factors as whether they see it as a gain or loss (loss aversion), who made the proposal (reactive devaluation), or what they believe about why the other party acted as he or she did (attribution theory) (Arrow et al. 1995; Mnookin, Peppet, and Tulumello 2000, 165–66; Allred 2000). *Loss aversion* describes the tendency of individuals to take risks to avoid a loss but to avoid risk when faced with a gain. This research suggests that how a proposed solution is packaged,[7] as a gain or as a loss, will significantly affect the likelihood of its acceptance. For example, in a dispute between neighbors about noise, a proposal that the man upstairs stop playing music after ten o'clock may be seen by him as a loss and make him willing to risk litigation over the nuisance complaint. If, however, the proposal is framed as leaving him free to play music until ten without worrying about the reaction of the downstairs neighbor, he is likely to see it as a gain worth holding onto rather than risking a worse outcome in court.

*Reactive devaluation* describes the phenomenon that leads people to be suspicious of proposals when they are offered by someone seen as an "enemy" but to be accepting when the same proposal comes from someone who is trusted (Mnookin, Peppet, and Tulumello 2000, 165–66; Thompson and Nadler 2000; Arrow et al. 1995). The line of thinking seems to be, "That seems like an interesting idea, almost what I was going to propose, but my adversary is suggesting it, so it must be good for him. And if it is good for him, it must be bad for me."

*Attribution theory* suggests that whether people respond to a perceived offense with anger and blame may depend on the beliefs of the offended person about why

---

7. Some mediation texts refer to framing a proposal. We use the term "packaging" to avoid confusing "framing" and "reframing."

the offender acted as he or she did (Allred 2000). For example, someone cutting in on a line at the checkout counter is likely to be met with angry words, while someone who cuts in saying, "I'm so sorry, but I need to get home to my sick child" will be met with cooperation.

Mediators can improve their chances of avoiding these cognitive barriers that block resolution by using caucuses to float proposed solutions without attributing the solution to the adversary and by packaging proposals as gains for both sides.[8]

### Focusing on the Future

Often by the time parties get to mediation, they have become hostile and are more focused on who is to blame than on the problem and what to do in the future. Thus, the mediator's job, after gathering enough history to understand what brought the parties to the mediation table and why they may react in certain ways, is to redirect the parties' concern about blame and focus on what needs to happen now. Whereas in a trial the focus is on proving facts and assessing blame for past behavior and events, in bioethics mediation the focus is on the present and the future—on determining the parties' current goals and finding a solution to the dispute.

These are only some of the techniques used by mediators to help parties resolve their disputes. They can be powerful tools, so mediators should use them responsibly, remembering that the mediator's role is not to impose his or her ideas on the parties but to empower the parties by helping them explore solutions and choose the resolution that honors their goals, values, and needs.

---

8. For an in-depth discussion of such barriers, see Arrow et al. 1995; Thompson and Nadler 2000.

# III

---

# CASE ANALYSES

*This part uses real cases to demonstrate the strengths and the weaknesses of the mediation process. The three cases analyzed here come from the files of the Montefiore Medical Center Bioethics Consultation Service. "Mr. Samuels's Case" (Chapter 6), "Mrs. Bates's Case" (Chapter 7), and "Mrs. Leonari's Case" (Chapter 8) tell the stories of three challenging mediations and the mediators' reflections on each case. The names have been changed and the medical histories altered to protect the privacy of the patients, families, and care providers. None of the stories, however, has been changed to heighten the service's successes or disguise its failures. Where memoranda are quoted, they reflect the actual text as closely as possible, while preserving the privacy of the participants.*

*It is important to understand that the order of interventions varies from case to case. Personalities affect the outcome as much as—often more than—do theories. Practice is influenced by factors that are extraneous to the case. So, for example, any conflict that begins to build before a major holiday, especially between Christmas and New Year's, when most doctors take time off, is doomed to stumble along without much resolution until the key attending physicians and consultants return from a long holiday. The immediate needs of the patient are addressed, but diagnostic tests are slow to be accomplished and difficult medical judgments tend to be postponed. Such is life in most teaching hospitals.*

*Reality shapes these narratives, as do power differentials, personalities, unaddressed discontents, and unrelated family crises; these are patients and families in conflict, and the unfolding narrative cannot be expected to move smoothly. The cases, commentaries, and discussions provide a valuable basis for thinking about the nature and composition of a bioethics mediation.*

# 6

## Mediation with a Competent Patient:
## Mr. Samuels's Case

### Background

Mr. Samuels was a 77-year-old man admitted to the medical center from home with end-stage emphysema. According to Dr. Peterman, a pulmonologist who had been his community doctor for several years, Mr. Samuels was a "Damon Runyon-esque character"—an irascible man who never married, loved to gamble, and continued to smoke even after his health was threatened. Dr. Peterman treated him for emphysema for many years although the patient, despite a worsening condition, refused to stop smoking, use his oxygen, or take his medications regularly.

One year before the mediation of his case, Mr. Samuels was hospitalized in acute respiratory failure. He had had trouble breathing, he had widely disseminated infection in his blood (sepsis), and he had recently exhibited severe liver damage. At that time he was put on a ventilator. With treatment, he improved and was successfully weaned from the ventilator, but after he returned home, he deteriorated rapidly. At about this time, his companion of 40 years, Dorothy Langer, gave up her apartment and moved in with him. She referred to herself as his common-law wife. Once a very active woman, she now suffered with severe arthritis and was compelled to use a walker.

A few months later, Mr. Samuels complained of pain in his side and back, which Dr. Peterman initially thought was due to fractured ribs caused by several falls. Eventually Mr. Samuels was admitted to the hospital with severe back pain; an MRI showed possible metastases and a CT scan showed extensive osteoporosis. He was managed with medications, and although a bone biopsy was recommended, it was not done. The test requires that a patient lie on his stomach, which Mr. Samuels was unable to do because of his pulmonary compromise. He was put on a ventilator and there was a discussion about the possibility that he might not come off. Mr. Samuels was very clear that he did not want to live like that. Finally, however, a biopsy showed no cancer and he was again weaned from the ventilator. At that time, Mr. Samuels appointed Ms. Langer as his health care proxy.

Subsequently, Mr. Samuels experienced more respiratory problems that led to a readmission to the pulmonary intensive care unit (PICU). He suffered a cardiac arrest and was put back on the ventilator, from which it was not possible to wean him.

Mr. Samuels, however, began asking to be extubated, or removed from the ventilator, clearly articulating his understanding that removal might very well lead to his death. Ten days after the intubation, a tracheostomy was recommended to make him more comfortable and perhaps permit him to speak. Mr. Samuels initially refused and again asked to be allowed to die; this was on a Friday. Dr. Peterman was concerned about proceeding without Ms. Langer and suggested waiting until Monday when he would again be on duty. During the weekend, Ms. Langer came in with her nephew, a doctor at another metropolitan hospital, and together they persuaded Mr. Samuels to consent to the procedure.

Throughout this period, there had been numerous discussions with Dr. Peterman and other caregivers about the consequences of extubation and Mr. Samuels had been consistent and clear about his wish to die. At one point, Dr. Peterman wrote on a piece of paper, "You want to die" and "You want to live." The patient signed his name under the first sentence. Ms. Langer was vehemently opposed to extubation and insisted that Mr. Samuels did not know what he wanted. She was far from certain that he wanted to die. She believed that he was simply depressed. At this point Dr. Peterman asked for a bioethics mediation.

The first step the mediator took, after meeting with the care team, was to ask for a consultation with a psychiatrist from Geriatric Psychiatry. Dr. Garrison conducted a psychiatric evaluation and found Mr. Samuels to be capacitated and appropriately depressed about his situation. In her opinion, it would be unethical to give him psychotropic medicine to combat depression for the sole purpose of changing his mind about extubation. The risk manager, Ms. Torrent, supported the hospital's honoring the patient's request.

The mediator met with Dr. Peterman and several members of the care team, after which she and Dr. Peterman met for an extended discussion with Ms. Langer. Ms. Langer was quite desperate and had not been available to approaches by Dr. Peterman or the social worker assigned to the case. She accused Dr. Peterman of trying to influence Mr. Samuels to die and yelled that he should stay away from him. She said that Mr. Samuels was being selfish, thinking only of himself. She also expressed concern about the location of Mr. Samuels's money and the disposition of the apartment. Furthermore, she said, she had spoken with someone in the Patient Relations Department, complaining about what the hospital was doing to Mr. Samuels and suggesting she might hire an attorney. Dr. Peterman told Ms. Langer that Mr. Samuels was very concerned about her well-being and had asked for the name of an attorney who could help him make a will.

Shortly thereafter, the mediator met with Mr. Samuels who, at one point, nodded that he wanted to die and, at another point, that he did not.

Mrs. Feather, a supervising social worker, met with Ms. Langer for an extended discussion about Mr. Samuels's condition, prognosis, and wishes, as well as Ms. Langer's own needs. Ms. Langer described her background and provided some insights into her current situation. She had been a fashion model, and her orthopedic problems requiring the use of a walker were very distressing to her. Her marriage had ended in a messy, painful divorce and she was distanced from her only child, a son who was a pediatrician in Florida. Ms. Langer expressed her great fear of being alone, especially at night, and her inability to envision anything to live for if Mr. Samuels died. She acknowledged that perhaps it was she who was being somewhat selfish in clinging to Mr. Samuels. She consented to Mrs. Feather's calling her son and exploring the possibility of her going to Florida to live with him and her two grandchildren. She also revealed that she had a history of psychiatric illnesses and, on her own, called a psychiatrist from liaison psychiatry for help; he agreed to provide ongoing psychiatric treatment.

Previously, a nurse from the PICU had asked this psychiatrist, Dr. Burton, to see Mr. Samuels. By the time Dr. Burton met with Mr. Samuels, he had become less certain that he wanted to die and had asked the staff to explore other options, including his going home on the ventilator. Ms. Langer insisted that a feeding tube, also under consideration, would be a poor choice for Mr. Samuels because food was so important to him, and a speech-and-swallowing consult was scheduled to diagnose swallowing problems. At this point most staff thought that the resolution would be a transfer to a nursing home.

After a week of consultation and patient vacillation, Dr. Peterman and the bioethics consultant posed several questions to Mr. Samuels about future care options. Mr. Samuels was now consistent, expressing clearly that he wanted to be disconnected from the ventilator and that he accepted that the likely consequence would be death. In fact, he mouthed that he wanted to die and indicated with unequivocal hand gestures that he wanted his life-support cut off. He rejected any option that included remaining attached to the ventilator—including being transferred to a nursing home or returning home to be cared for by Ms. Langer and home health aides. Despite his expressed desires in private conversations, Ms. Langer continued to claim that Mr. Samuels did not want to die and would like to be cared for at home. And when questioned in Ms. Langer's presence, he did sometimes change his statements.

After meeting briefly with Mr. Samuels, the care team convened to discuss a plan of care. In addition to Dr. Peterman and the mediator, the "team" included a representative from Risk Management, two social workers, and two pulmonary residents.

The mediator opened the discussion by reminding all of the team that decisions to terminate life-sustaining treatment are inherently accompanied by ambivalence. Mr. Samuels's apparent indecision and Ms. Langer's expressions of fear and anxiety were natural. Nevertheless, it was essential that all participants in the decision-making process concur that Mr. Samuels was now clear and that his expressed interests and his unambivalent wishes were best served by disconnecting him from the ventilator. While no member at the meeting dissented, there remained some lingering uncertainty about whether disconnecting the ventilator would result in Mr. Samuels's death.

The team decided to pursue the following course of action: First, Mr. Samuels would have another psychiatric evaluation to establish, finally, his capacity to make a decision about his care and about his death. Second, Ms. Langer would receive grief counseling. Finally, one week from the meeting, Mr. Samuels's situation would be revisited. If all remained the same (especially his desire to end his present suffering), the ventilator would be disconnected. If he were unable to breathe on his own, comfort care and morphine would be provided.

After the meeting, Dr. Peterman and the mediator discussed the plan with Mr. Samuels and Ms. Langer. They made it clear that in one week the situation would be reevaluated and that if Mr. Samuels still wished to be disconnected from the ventilator at that time, his wishes would be respected. In the meantime, the team hoped, Ms. Langer would be able to come to some sort of peace with the possibility of his death. The mediator called in a special social work supervisor with experience in bereavement counseling. This person agreed to meet with Ms. Langer daily for the week that the plan was in progress. Assured that his wishes would be respected, Mr. Samuels agreed to the one-week delay.

The psychiatrist reported that Mr. Samuels was aware of his condition and clear and consistent about his wants. The final discussion a week later confirmed that Mr. Samuels was ready to have his ventilator disconnected. He said good-bye to Ms. Langer, who went back to their apartment, where her son awaited her. (Ms. Langer had used the week to talk with her son and arrange for him to come to be with her when the extubation took place.) The resident started an intravenous line so that morphine could be provided when needed.

At this point, a new question arose, and the mediator and Dr. Peterman engaged in a lively discussion about the administration of morphine. The mediator questioned when morphine would be given; perhaps at the outset? Dr. Peterman replied no, that morphine would be provided when the patient indicated discomfort. He canceled all plans for the remainder of the day. Then he disconnected the ventilator and sat down next to the bed to monitor Mr. Samuels's condition. Twenty minutes later, Mr. Samuels started to squirm. When asked if he was uncomfortable, he nodded yes. Morphine was administered. Two hours later, when Mr. Samuels still seemed comfortable but was no longer aware, Dr. Peterman and the mediator left. A constant shift of nurses stayed by Mr. Samuels's bed; he died 43 hours later.

## Analysis

The mediator's role in Mr. Samuels's case was sixfold.[1]

1. *Supporting the patient.* It was important that the mediator not ask Mr. Samuels the same question continuously ("Do you want to terminate life supports?") so that he would feel he had to beg for support for his decision. Once capacity is established and clinical depression is ruled out, the role of the mediator is to capture and amplify the voice of the patient. The patient must be told that he has been heard, that his wishes will be respected, and that there is a plan to implement his choice. This plan represents a "principled resolution" (see box, p. 111), based on his status as a competent and fully informed patient who has chosen to refuse care and accept death.

2. *Exploring all options.* The mediator had to consider whether it would be worth delaying the termination of life support for a few days to help Ms. Langer prepare for the inevitability of Mr. Samuels's death. If such a delay would not be harmful to the patient and was acceptable to him, it might help his partner and thus also be in his interest. The determinative factor in this decision was how the delay would affect the patient and whether he would agree. If remaining on the ventilator, even for a few days, would significantly increase Mr. Samuels's physical or ex-

---

1. This analysis is based on extensive comments from Professor Barbara Swartz.

istential suffering, such a plan would be difficult to justify. If, however, appropriate medication and the assurance of a time-certain plan for extubation would enable Mr. Samuels to tolerate a few more days on the ventilator to promote Ms. Langer's comfort, her needs might assume greater weight ethically. End-of-life care requires treating the patient in the context of family and beloved others.

3. *Determining who would be at the table.*  The staff of the PICU was very attached to Mr. Samuels. He had been there for almost three months and had been cared for by every nurse and house staff officer who had rotated through the unit. He had become part of the family that lives and works together in the PICU; everyone wanted to respect his wishes and not see him suffer. This level of concern among the staff was not crucial to the practical or ethical outcome of the case but it underlined the importance of including the staff in the decision-making process.

Although they did not necessarily like her, staff were also attached to Ms. Langer. They respected the fact that she was there every day and sat by the bedside. They respected the positions that she took in fighting for Mr. Samuels's life. They had sympathy for her panic at being left alone; they wanted to support her. Some of the consultants had assumed the care of Ms. Langer, seeing her as a patient to whom they owed separate and individual obligations of care. This sense of obligation to Ms. Langer became a factor in how care providers assessed their roles and responsibilities.

As the plan developed, the mediator held frequent conferences with the staff to keep them up-to-date on Mr. Samuels's position, on the state of the negotiations, and on the evolution of a plan. She explained that while she was committed to Mr. Samuels's support she was equally committed to ensuring that Ms. Langer not be left out of the circle of concern. All agreed. Many staff had suggestions for how to talk to and deal with both Mr. Samuels and Ms. Langer. The developing timetable was discussed and all staff were asked if they wanted, particularly, to be excluded from the staffing during the extubation. No one took this option. All were comfortable with the patient's decision and all were comfortable being part of the process.

4. *Disaggregating the issues and bringing clarity to complex discussions.*  Two issues, in sequence, challenged the team: the first was Ms. Langer's inability to face the fact of Mr. Samuels's impending death and the second was Dr. Peterman's reluctance to use morphine in the initial stages of extubation.

With regard to the first, the mediator worked slowly but consistently to reiterate the right of a decisionally capable patient to choose to refuse care and accept death. This principle was not unknown to the staff, but the issues of prognosis and clinical depression encouraged some staff to question the capacitated basis of Mr. Samuels's decision and his ability to confront the awesome choice. Although there had been some psychiatric evaluation over the months of Mr. Samuels's stay in the PICU, the psychiatric consultant requested by the mediator was particularly skilled in geriatric care and was very comfortable with the issue of choosing death. His note in the chart that the patient was "appropriately depressed" by the prospect of death was extremely helpful to the staff.

The mediator, acting in the role of consultant within the mediation process, insisted that Mr. Samuels be told that his wishes had been heard and his request would be honored. She then explained to him that the staff would like some time to work with Ms. Langer to help her be ready for his extubation and confirmed that this step would be acceptable to him. In complex multiparty mediation there is some ethical responsibility to all of the parties, including the staff and the family. The patient is the primary focus but others have interests, too, that need to be isolated and addressed, if at all possible.

Finally, whether and when morphine would be administered was an issue between the mediator and Dr. Peterman, who was determined not to use morphine until he deemed it necessary. The mediator was very concerned about Mr. Samuels's comfort but was reassured that Dr. Peterman would be there and would respond immediately. Since this was a difficult case for Dr. Peterman, who hates to "lose" a patient, the mediator accepted his stance. Had the physician objected to the use of morphine or set rigid rules, the mediator would have been faced with a different set of issues that might have required triggering a broader discussion with other pulmonologists or with the palliative care team. This part of the mediation called for the mediator to be prepared to change hypotheses.

Mr. Samuels's case illustrates the fact that the mediator needs to be the "advocate for the plan." Resolution and follow-up may be as difficult in the medical setting as the initial fact gathering and development of options. Implementing a plan, especially one that facilitates the death of a patient, challenges the instinct and training of many medical professionals.

5. *Providing ongoing education about the principles and practices involved in the case.* In addition to engaging in lengthy discussions with the staff, the mediator left long notes in the chart that provided the rationale for such concepts as "decision-specific capacity" and the right of the patient to choose death not as a form of suicide but as a reflection of capacity. These notes were especially helpful to staff members who had not been at the team discussions.

**6.** *Advocating for the "principled resolution."* The mediator assumed the role of advocate for the patient's plan to discontinue care once it was clear that this was an informed and voluntary choice that was not the product of clinical depression. Advocacy, however, needed to occur in the frame of the ethical obligations not to abandon Ms. Langer and to help her prepare for the advent of Mr. Samuels's death. This advocacy for fairness and the regard for the patient's beloved others is one aspect of bioethics mediation that differentiates it from other types of mediation. The mediator felt, as did the PICU staff, that Ms. Langer's inability to permit Mr. Samuels his desired outcome was an issue to be addressed in the context of putting together a care plan for Mr. Samuels. Had Mr. Samuels insisted on being extubated immediately, leaving the staff no time to work with Ms. Langer, his rights and the interest of Ms. Langer would have been in conflict and the staff would have had to choose to meet the patient's needs. But some negotiation with Mr. Samuels averted that direct collision.

In this case the roles of mediator, helping the parties to identify options for solution and choose among them, and consultant, identifying the "right" of the patient to choose death and working clearly toward that goal, were intertwined during all stages of the mediation. The mediator pursued the issues with the staff, the consultants, and Ms. Langer, confident that consensus could be reached. As it developed, Ms. Langer was simply implacable; she could not be persuaded that Mr. Samuels was truly making a decision to choose death. But as the staff and the patient moved toward consensus and additional supports were provided for Ms. Langer, a plan emerged that all could support.

# 7

## Mediation with a Dysfunctional Family: Mrs. Bates's Case

### Background

Mrs. Bates was a 75-year-old patient who was transferred to the medical center from a community hospital with the diagnosis of stenosis (narrowing of the cardiac valve). Her admission had followed a series of four visits to the Emergency Room of the hospital near her home, where she had gone to seek help for difficulty in breathing. She arrived at the medical center with a guarded cardiac prognosis and the label of "schizophrenia," though this characterization did not come up in the mediation and seemed irrelevant to the issues under discussion.[1]

The patient was alert and able to make the decision to transfer from the community hospital and, after admission, the subsequent decisions to undergo surgery. She had appointed a daughter, one of five children, as her health care agent, or proxy. She had also executed a living will that stated that it would take effect if there were a "terminal condition." At the medical center she underwent two surgeries. She did well following the first, to replace the aortic valve, and was considered for discharge but developed a deep infection leading to heart block and needed a second surgery to implant a pacemaker. The atrial lead then became dislodged and the patient became hypotensive and was returned to surgery for repair of the mitral valve. She also developed an infection on her tricuspid valve, for which she was treated with antibiotics; she entered renal failure, for which she was started on peritoneal dialysis. The medical team was not certain that the infection could be controlled with antibiotic use but had agreed that further surgery was not an option. Soon after the start of the dialysis treatments, the patient experienced a car-

---

1. Note that psychiatric labels often muddy already turbulent waters by suggesting issues of decisional incapacity. In this case, as in many others, the label did not present relevant material.

diac arrest and was placed on a ventilator. The patient's daughter, acting as her mother's health care agent, requested a do not resuscitate (DNR) order; the cardiac surgeon was opposed to writing the order. To resolve the impasse, the clinical care coordinator (CCC), a nurse in the Cardiac Intensive Care Unit, requested a bioethics consultation.

At the time of the initial consult, Mrs. Bates was intermittently "somewhat alert." She had been refractory to weaning from the ventilator and had been labeled "vent dependent." The bioethics mediator was not able to meet first with the medical team alone. Present at the initial meeting were the patient's daughter, the daughter's husband, the cardiac surgeon, the cardiac surgical fellow, the bioethics mediator, and an experienced mediator on sabbatical with the consult service.

The bioethics mediator started the meeting by introducing herself and the process. She explained who she was, that she worked for the hospital as chairperson of the Ethics Committee and director of the Division of Bioethics, and that her role in this case was to see whether any agreement could be reached on the plan of care. She then asked for a review of the medical facts.

The cardiac surgeon stated at the outset that the meeting could be short, for he had determined that the patient was not "terminal" and in fact was getting better. The CCC, however, did not share this judgment.

After the facts had been presented, the mediator asked the daughter to state what she had learned in discussions with her mother and why she felt that her mother would want a DNR order at this time.

The daughter, clearly under stress, began quite strongly. In discussions, she reported, her mother had been very clear that if she had a diminished quality of life from her cardiac disease and from chronic obstructive pulmonary disease, which continued to worsen in response to her continued smoking, she would not want to have life-sustaining care continued. She had been clear, too, the daughter stated, that she did not want to "die twice"; if she arrested she did not want to be resuscitated. As a devout Evangelical Christian, Mrs. Bates felt that if she experienced a cardiac arrest, it was her time to die and she did not want to act against what she saw as a divine verdict. The daughter pointed out that these wishes, though voiced in the context of a "terminal condition," were, in general, what her mother wanted to guide her care. She had had many discussions with her mother on this issue and the message had been consistent.

As soon as the daughter finished, her husband and the surgeon attacked her. Her husband stated, and the surgeon agreed, that a DNR order would lessen the amount and the quality of care that the patient would receive and might compromise her chances of recovery. The husband explained that he was speaking from experience. His father had been in the hospital recently and the family had fought to get him the most aggressive care. The husband intimated that the patient's daughter was morally inadequate and not sufficiently loving and protective of her mother if she did not do the same. He equated a DNR order with a do-not-treat order and suggested that by signing such an order she was abandoning her mother. The daughter stood fast in her position for a while and then folded under the assault of the two men.

The dynamic of the conversation in the mediation meeting was extremely unbalanced and the atmosphere was tense. The mediator backed off, reluctant to intervene in the complex relationships of dependence and abuse that seemed to characterize the daughter-husband and daughter-surgeon relationships. But once the daughter withdrew her support for a DNR order, the mediator reentered the discussion, emphasizing that decisions about ethical issues are grounded in the medical status of the moment and can and should be revisited as the status of the patient evolves.

The chart note, filed on the consultation report form, stated that the daughter had agreed "for the moment not to insist on the DNR but that, should her mom take a turn for the worse, she would want this decision reconsidered [and] . . . if the patient continues to improve the plan is ethically supportable. If the patient deteriorates, her wishes and those of her proxy should be respected and a DNR written, [for] . . . time is the ally of an ethical plan."

A week after the meeting, the CCC called the mediator to report that the patient was yet weaker and less responsive. The mediator asked her to call the daughter, report this finding, and confirm that she was still comfortable with a care plan that did not include a DNR order. The CCC made this call and, shortly thereafter, the daughter called the surgeon to report that she was being harassed by the CCC. The surgeon then called the CCC, who called the mediator. The mediator sent an e-mail message to the surgeon to clarify that the call to the daughter had been at the request of the mediator pursuant to the notion that the conclusion of the prior mediation had identified a time-limited solution that should be reevaluated as the status of the patient changed.

Three days later the surgeon called the mediator to state that the patient had taken a turn for the worse and he was, in consultation with the daughter, writing a DNR order.

## Analysis

After this case, the following issues were identified by the visiting mediator, who sat in on the mediation (with full agreement of all parties).[2]

1. *The physician's judgment of the medical status of the patient.*  The physician's judgment would seem to be the natural grounding for any discussion about the ethical plan of care. Yet in this case one could argue that the physician's judgment was not necessarily a reliable basis for patient evaluation and decision making. Surgeons are particularly committed to supporting their patients through the hard times that follow the complicated course of recovery from multiple surgeries. They hate to lose. Moreover, any death within 30 days of surgery must be reported to the medical examiner's office. Such reports almost never result in any action, but the process is distasteful to most surgeons. The CCC seemed more objective, yet when conflicts of interest exist, and fixed prospective payment and limited reimbursement conflict with a plan of care with little prospect of success, the CCC's responsibility for length-of-stay and discharge planning must be factored into interpretations of medical advice. The CCC in this case might have seen Mrs. Bates as a vent-dependent patient who would greatly exceed her length of stay and thereby lose money for the hospital and tarnish the CCC's record.

2. *The daughter's statements about her mother's conversations and wishes.*  The daughter was very specific about her mother's wishes and quoted conversations in detail and with the sort of language that rings true to discussions with medically unsophisticated patients and families. The mediator had never heard of the concept of not wanting to "die twice" and therefore accorded it great weight.

3. *The living will.*  Many advance directive documents are filled out carelessly at the instigation of some institutional official. Many do not reflect the real wishes of the patient. Yet they may be the best evidence available of the personal values of the patient. A written document that deals with transplantation and autopsy, as this one did, and where the other choices are consistent, has a great deal of force. In general, written documents need to be interpreted in the light of the patient's condition and the other aspects of the patient's personality that emerge in discussion with the family. This document supported and reinforced the statements of the daughter. Furthermore, the question of whether a patient is "terminal" is the trigger question

---

2. We are grateful to Professor Barbara Swartz for suggesting these categories.

for most living wills, and, as this case demonstrates, is a category that requires a level of interpretation that generally renders it counterproductive in discussion.

4. *Family dynamics.* Responding to the bullying and intimidating nature of the husband was an issue in this mediation. His attitude was threatening, his words harsh, and his behavior overbearing and hostile. The way the couple communicated was clearly not limited to this circumstance. It was not inconceivable that this was a physically abusive relationship and if it was, the mediator had to take care not to provoke the man further against his wife. Dysfunctional modes of communication established in nonstressful times are likely to be even more pronounced under stress. In this case the bullying husband was supported by the physician.

In standard family mediation, when one of the parties begins bullying the other, most mediators would recognize their obligation to explore whether mediation is the best means of resolving the conflict. Although to be "transparent" about the problem in a joint session may risk reinforcing the power differential, in a private caucus with the less powerful party, the mediator could be open about the possibility that if the power differential cannot be overcome, mediation might be impossible. In the case of Mrs. Bates, however, this strategy was not an option. First, the mediation could not be postponed, since a decision was required to establish the patient's care plan. Second, the power relationships were an established feature of the parties' modes of interacting.

The dynamics of the family, or at least those of the patient's daughter and her husband, were bound to defeat the daughter-proxy in her goal of following her mother's wishes as she understood them. Intervention by the mediator risked making matters worse, interrupting the basis of the doctor-proxy relationship that existed, and exacerbating the tension between the husband and the wife. Also, it was the perception of the mediator, based on a review of the chart and the statements of the members of the care team, that this was a dying patient. The patient's course could have changed rapidly, but it was more, rather than less, likely that the patient was on a path to death. If the wishes of the daughter, reflecting the values of her mother, were supported and if the patient died, the daughter would be blamed by her husband, and perhaps by the rest of her family, as the cause of death. The mediator was loath to place this burden on the daughter. Work on the doctor-proxy relationship has demonstrated that the proxy must not only factor in the interests and wishes of the patient but must also protect his or her place in the constellation of the family. The proxy has his or her own interests to shield and the mediator must not undercut this impulse (Symposium 1999).

As Tia Powell (1999) so eloquently demonstrates, the fact that one person has been appointed as the legal proxy does not dispense with the complexity of family choice. The dynamics of the family are such that if the patient is not suffering, his or her wishes must sometimes be subordinated, at least temporarily, to the emotional needs of the family members, for they must live with the solution and the consequences after the patient dies.

5. *Patient's pain and suffering.*   This patient was not experiencing pain. She was sufficiently debilitated and sufficiently sedated that she was not fighting the ventilator and seemed not to be agitated. Because pain is an ethical issue, not just a medical one, if the patient had been in pain the equities of the situation would have been different. But she was, to the best of the caregivers' ability to judge, not in pain, and the daughter had to decide what was good for her mother in the context of her own life, at that moment and in the future. Family members, like the daughter in this case, often decide in ways that will permit them to face the future without the patient and with the surviving relatives.

If the patient were suffering, then the role of the mediator would be bounded much more narrowly by the medical interests of the patient. Whereas bioethics mediation is patient-centered, and must take account of patient suffering, it is also family-centered and must help the family members live with each other after the death, recovery, revival, or disability of the patient.

As with any mediation, the agenda for the mediator is determined by the immediacy of the situation and by the characteristics of the drama. The mediator needs to approach the meetings with family and staff with a notion of the issues (a working hypothesis) and some rough order of priority of the issues to be discussed, all subject to emendation as the narrative unfolds. In an end-of-life mediation the interests of the patient in a realistic care plan that balances the burdens and benefits of the treatment and in a death without unnecessary pain and suffering are paramount.

These issues, again, are no different from the sort of issue, such as property, custody, and visiting schedules, a mediator might face in any situation of family conflict. In every case, mediation must be grounded by rules, principles, public policy, and the reality of the family dynamics.

One final role of the mediator, as illustrated in this case, is to help the family bear the burden of difficult decisions. There is a huge difference, for example, between asking a family member whether he or she wants to sign a DNR order for the patient and suggesting that such an order is the appropriate care plan. With the former, many family members feel that they have signed a "death warrant." With the latter, if the family accepts the plan, the physician can carry the onus of the decision. For family members there is a fine line, to which mediators must be sensitive, between bearing the burden of the decision and feeling disempowered.

# 8

## A Complex Mediation with a Large and Involved Family: Mrs. Leonari's Case

### Background

The first sign that a conflict was brewing was a flurry of e-mail messages. One from an administrator high up in the organization went to a hospital vice president. The note stated that the family of a patient was unhappy with the care the patient was receiving in the Surgical Intensive Care Unit (SICU). A second e-mail message, between the same parties, indicated that the two surgeons in charge of the unit were in dispute about the care the patient should receive. A third message, a response from the vice president with the previous e-mail correspondence attached, suggested that the Bioethics Consultation Service be called into the case.

On that same day, the nursing supervisor in the SICU called the bioethics mediators for the hospital, requesting a bioethics consultation. The reason provided for the request, a bioethics issue, was that the family was interfering with the appropriate care for the patient and the interests of the patient were imperiled.

The two bioethics mediators who picked up the case, Andy Purdure and Virginia Lieland, agreed that a principled frame for the problem would probably be that the patient's well-being was in jeopardy and that the obligation of the staff to pursue the best interest of the patient, a principle called "beneficence," was threatened. As a matter of course the ethical obligation of the staff to care for the present needs of the patient defines appropriate care. Family interference with the standard of care is always troubling.

A second bioethics issue inherent in the initial narrative was the allocation of scarce resources. A bed in the SICU is a scarce resource that must be allocated fairly and is generally assigned according to the principle of triage—a bed to that person who can benefit the most, who is neither too sick to benefit nor too healthy to justify this level of care. The staff in an intensive care unit is also a scarce resource. A patient's family that is too demanding and takes up a disproportionate amount of time and energy deprives other patients of the care that they require.

This bioethics mediation team usually begins the mediation process by speaking with the referring person, reviewing the chart, and convening all of the care providers. In general, this initial meeting comprises four to six staff members who brief one or more of the mediation team on the case, describe the medical condition of the patient (history, diagnosis, prognosis), relate the interactions with the family, and express whatever emotions are clouding the creation of a successful and shared plan of care for the patient. This case was unusual from the start; 18 staff members gathered in one of the empty rooms of the SICU. Participants included the two surgeons in charge of the unit, the supervising nurse and six nurses from the unit, two physician assistants, the two surgical fellows, one social worker, and four house staff and medical students. The emotional maelstrom was immediately apparent, indeed overwhelming.

The first step in any classical mediation, "setting the stage," or arranging the participants around a table, is rarely possible in bioethics mediations and was not possible in this case. Staff rolled chairs over from the nurses' station, the bank of monitoring machines, the other patient rooms, and the adjoining medical service; three or four sat on the empty bed; others leaned against the windowsill. One of the surgeons sat but the other one, concerned about the care of another patient who was in crisis, stood in the door to have a clear view of a particular monitor that he had turned to be visible from the doorway.

Mr. Purdure and Ms. Lieland began by using their standard protocol: introducing themselves as bioethics consultants and mediators and asking the person who called the consult to explain why in this case she had thought that there was an ethical problem. The supervising nurse explained that the nursing staff was so distraught over the behavior of this family and so fearful of them because of their complaints to supervisors and administrators that they were reluctant to care for the patient; the staff continued to provide excellent care, she hastened to assure everyone, but she was concerned that this family's behavior was on the verge of compromising the patient's care.

Drs. Kibbe and Lordson, jointly in charge of the case, then explained that, indeed, there was no difference between them in their evaluation of this case and in their plan for managing the patient. The rumor of conflict between the surgeons had originated, they explained, not in disagreements about the care of the patient but rather in miscommunication about the management of the family. The facts, Dr. Kibbe explained, were as follows: on the Monday morning preceding this first bioethics meeting, the supervising nurse had arrived to find that Dr. Kibbe had written a note: "The family is only allowed to visit the patient between the hours of noon and eight p.m. and only for 10 minutes each hour." On her arrival at 8:00 a.m., she was accosted by the family and, because she had been absent for the weekend, she checked with Dr. Lordson, who stated, "I am in the middle of rounds. Do what you please with the family and we will discuss it later." Under pressure from the family, the nurse permitted them into the patient's room at 8:30.

The confrontation had its roots in the family's use of cell phones in the patient's room. They had been warned time and again that cell phones might interfere with the patient monitors. After one of the daughters was "caught" three times talking on a cell phone in the patient's room, Dr. Kibbe set the limit: the family would be able to visit the patient for only ten minutes an hour between noon and 8:00 p.m. They were to be barred from visiting at any other time. Clearly the family, and not the patient, was the focus of the conflict.

Mr. Purdure asked the surgical fellow in the unit to provide a brief medical history of the case. At the time of the meeting, the patient, Mrs. Leonari, had been in the SICU for over three months. She had been stricken with pancreatitis—rather like being hit by lightning—had quickly progressed to multisystem organ failure, had been brought to surgery twice, and appeared now to have a colonic fistula that would likely involve additional surgery. At the moment, the patient was dependent on ventilatory support and probably not experiencing any pain. The surgical fellow noted that the patient appeared not to recognize or respond to family and staff, although some of the family members felt otherwise and asserted their opinions clearly when challenged.

The surgical fellow's report was a straightforward recitation of the devastation that pancreatitis creates. At the moment the patient was improving slightly, but 98 percent of the way to real stability was yet to be traversed. And, were the patient to become stable, she would face many more months in a rehabilitation facility before she might be able to negotiate a return home. The best scenario was more months in the SICU, perhaps more surgery, and if all went without further complication, an extended stay in rehabilitation—a guarded and grim prognosis.

Ms. Lieland then asked about the family and the following facts emerged. This was a Sicilian American family with five grown children, three daughters and two sons, who had immigrated to the United States in the 1960s. They had all prospered, some had attended college, others had entered businesses, and all had established flourishing careers. Three of them were involved in politics, at the local, state, and national levels, and paraded their political contacts whenever challenged by staff.

All of the patient's children had numerous, mainly small, children of their own at home. Most of the nurses and the medical staff saw this family as a devoted group who loved their mother with passion and who were disoriented by her sudden disappearance from their lives. This was a woman who made her own pasta sauce and pasta every weekend and had at least 20 of the family for dinner every Sunday. She offered food, advice, support, love, comfort, and structure to a family who had come together to this new land and succeeded beyond their dreams. This was not just the mother; this was the leader of the tribe.

Now the family was engaged in what they perceived to be the fierce pursuit of their mother's interests. They had explained to the supervising nurse that their mother had always done everything for the family and that now, when she needed them, they intended to be there for her. Their interpretation of this commitment was translated into staying with the patient day and night throughout the week. Indeed, two of the daughters had gone on reduced work schedules at their jobs and were running back and forth between houses, offices, and hospital. The children were convinced that their mother knew that they were there and that she experienced their abandonment when they were absent. They were all devout Roman Catholics who believed that saying prayers with their mother was one of the important elements in her recovery. The family began early in the morning saying prayers, stroking the patient's forehead and hands, bathing her gently with a damp cloth, smoothing her bed covers, and straightening her hospital gown.

The family was extremely solicitous for the staff and regularly brought them pastries, fruit, and multiple cups of coffee. They tried to be generous with all but always singled out some for particular praise. Some of the staff commented that this was a remarkable family, mutually supportive, loving, caring, and well organized. They were described as "doing the best they know how given the terrible condition of the patient." Dr. Kibbe suggested that these adult and very competent children of the patient were all infantilized by their status as children, albeit grown and largely in their thirties and forties, without the emotional and moral center that their mother provided. The patient's husband was devastated by her illness and appeared to grant leadership in staff relationships to the oldest of the children, Mrs. Cotrelli and Mrs. Dominick.

But this was only half the story. Other staff experienced the family as aggressive, intrusive, meddling, and threatening. Indeed, on one occasion when a tube had been temporarily closed by one of the bed wheels, a daughter threatened to murder the nurse if she were not more careful. The incident that had preceded the latest crisis had been the complaint by Mrs. Cotrelli, one of the patient's daughters, about the behavior of one nurse named Patti. Mrs. Cotrelli had reported to the supervisor that the nurse was rough and uncaring; Patti, when confronted with the family's displeasure, had reacted with outrage. She stated that she had cared for the patient with unfailing skill and was furious that the family had complained about the care.

As soon as one of the physicians or nurses entered the room the family bombarded him or her with questions. If there was any discrepancy in the answers provided, they pounced on another physician, physician assistant, or nurse to resolve what they saw as a conflict. When criticized for asking too many questions, they began to keep a notebook with responses that the family members who visited subsequently might read for the up-to-the-minute data on the status of their mother. Some of the staff understood this tactic as an accommodation to the needs of the staff and others saw it as preparing a record for later attack.

And all the staff resented the family's flouting of unit rules, such as no use of cell phones in the rooms of the patients, especially since they had been told repeatedly that the use of cell phones could interfere with the monitoring equipment. To the staff, the family's continued use of cell phones was sneaky and in disregard for the welfare of the patients, and they were unmoved by the explanation that the daughters had to use cell phones to keep in touch with small children at home—they should have left the unit for that.

Tempers were short, understanding was limited, and emotions were aroused. The visiting hours rule had been articulated on a Sunday, implemented the following Monday, affirmed on Tuesday, and intermittently disregarded by the family since then. The bioethics mediators entered the case on the Thursday following the promulgation of the rule.

At the conclusion of the meeting with the staff, the mediators stated that they would proceed to meet with the family members and would report back to the staff if compromise seemed possible.

The SICU is one of the critical care units in the hospital. Its staff is specially trained to make decisions about patient care in consultation with, but not under the authority of, the operating surgeon. This rule is variable, however, given the power and prestige of the patient's primary surgeon. In the vast majority of cases, including this one, the SICU team plans for and directs patient care. In addition, Dr. Kibbe was also the one who had performed the most recent operation on the patient.

The rules in the SICU state that visiting hours are 24 hours a day. The nurses had lobbied hard for this change from the previous policy, which had stipulated fixed visiting hours from 11:00 a.m. to 1:00 p.m. and from 6:00 p.m. to 8:00 p.m., because these set hours had excluded many family members and friends who had inflexible work schedules. In an effort to accommodate family needs, the rules had been changed. But until this case, no one had ever interpreted the rule literally to mean that the family could be there 24 hours a day, seven days a week.

The two mediators entered the patient's room and introduced themselves to Mrs. Cotrelli and Mrs. Dominick. They explained the Bioethics Consultation Service and their roles in identifying bioethics issues and helping to resolve bioethics conflicts. They also explained their roles in mediating disputes in the hospital, pointing out that they were employed by the hospital and therefore were not independent mediators.

During this time the daughters were sitting by their mother's bed, stroking her arms and saying prayers. They came to the side of the room to talk and they and the mediators pulled chairs in a circle. The mediators explained that they had just completed talking with the staff as a way of trying to understand the history of the present situation. They stated that the staff were very concerned that the family's constant presence in the unit was a disrupting factor in the care of the patient. They also explained that some staff felt threatened by what they perceived as the family's belligerent behavior and were very upset that the family would continue to use cell phones when clearly asked numerous times to refrain. They wanted to understand, from the perspective of the family, what had occurred.

The older daughter, Mrs. Cotrelli, began, "Our mom devoted her life to us and now she needs us and we expect to be here for her every moment of the day. She deserves no less. . . . We never interfere with care and we always leave when the nurses ask. . . . They are jealous that we love her so much and no one loves them like this." The two daughters stated that they were very pleased with the care and denied any problems with the staff, with the exception of one nurse who they felt was not properly responsive to their mother and did not bathe and care for her appropriately.

Ms. Lieland stated that the staff agreed unanimously that the family was interfering with the care of their mother. The daughters expressed shock and dismay and asked for help in ameliorating the situation.

Mr. Purdure suggested that they meet soon with some other members of the family, especially Mr. Leonari—the patient's husband—and try to forge some agreement that would help the family and the staff, locked in this forced togetherness, to get along. He especially requested that Mrs. Cotrelli invite her husband, who was a physician at this hospital, to join the discussion. The sisters agreed and asked that a meeting be set for that afternoon at five o'clock. It was known to Mr. Purdure, but not to the family, that this physician, son-in-law of the patient, had stated to the surgeon that he thought that the family would be helped by the setting of some boundaries. "Too much freedom was hard for them to handle," he had said.

At five Ms. Lieland and Mr. Purdure returned to the patient's room and found the two sisters and the husband of one of them, Mr. Dominick, a lawyer; neither the patient's husband nor Dr. Cotrelli was present. Mr. Dominick introduced himself and stated that he had been appointed the spokesperson for the family and he would negotiate for them all. After much shouting by all three family members about the unfairness of the rules and the surgeon who had promulgated them, the three agreed to abide by the rules for the weekend if the beginning hour could be changed from noon to 10:00 a.m. and if there were no restrictions on the visiting hours for the patient's husband. The daughters stated that they were especially concerned about their father, who had taken this illness of his wife as a mortal threat to his being. They emphasized that because of the restrictions on the children's visiting, their father had been staying for longer hours, and they feared for his health. Nonetheless, they wanted him to be able to be there whenever he felt that he could. Whereas the daughters were reluctant to agree to anything, Mr. Dominick urged them to agree as a strategic move to calm the waters.

When Mr. Dominick asked who employed the mediators, they explained that they were paid by the hospital and that part of their task was to try to find some consensus about care plans and behavior when there were conflicts between and among staff, family, and patient. They explained that they were on the hospital payroll and therefore could not be considered neutral and independent mediators but that they did try nonetheless to listen to all parties and assist in the process of mediation. Sometimes, they explained, they were able to help and sometimes not. They offered to look for common ground.

An hour into the discussion the father joined the group. He seemed quite frail and was tearful. He stood by the bedside for a short moment and then arranged himself silently at the farthest corner of the room from the patient's bed.

Finally an agreement was forged and the mediators wrote it up as a chart note. After discussing the substance of the note with the family, they showed it to the nurses, who agreed generally that it was an improvement but were reluctant to commit to the unlimited hours for the husband. One nurse swayed the discussion by noting that the husband never stayed for long and was the easiest to handle. All agreed that Dr. Kibbe needed to approve the compromise before it became official.

The chart note stated:

> Consult requested by nurse supervisor to consult on the care of this patient, given a breakdown in communication with the family.
>
> Mr. Purdure and Ms. Lieland met with the staff on Thursday at 11 a.m. and with two daughters, and a son-in-law, Mr. Dominick, at 5 p.m. At 6 o'clock the patient's husband joined the discussion.
>
> Our goal is to forge a temporary consensus to quiet the strong feelings on both sides. The policy now in effect restricts visits to the hours between 10 a.m. and 8 p.m., and limits them to 10 minutes per hour.
>
> We suggest the following as a reasonable temporary compromise:
>
> 1. Rule limiting visits to 10 minutes/hour between noon and 8 p.m. remains in effect for Friday through Monday and applies to all visitors except the patient's husband.
> 2. Patient's husband may visit at will as long as all visitors, including the patient's husband, comply with the following conditions:
>    a. Use the intercom for clearance before each visit before entering
>    b. Do not interfere with any nursing care and leave when asked
> 3. On Tuesday morning at 11 the staff and family with these consultants will review the policy and the family's compliance and will consider rules for the future.
> 4. Acceptance of this plan must await approval by Dr. Kibbe or Dr. Lordson.

A copy of the note was given to the family members to share with others who were not present. That night Ms. Lieland sent the following e-mail message to Dr. Kibbe, who had originally ordered the restrictions. She felt that the staff's perspective had been presented to the family but that there had not been an equal opportunity to argue the family's feelings and position to the surgeon.

> TO: Dr. Kibbe
> FROM: Virginia Lieland
> RE: Thoughts over the night; 5:30 a.m.
>
> Needless to say you have seen the note that Andy Purdure and I left in the chart. I realized that I should have left a private note for you—thus this message.
>
> We spent time with Mrs. Cotrelli, Mrs. Dominick and her husband, and the patient's husband. I was impressed by all of the themes that had been raised yesterday morning. They are desperate at the loss of this person who has been the cen-

ter of the family. Mrs. Cotrelli, especially, feels this woman is her line to life and to meaning.

But, there is more. This is a very religious family, religious in a way that would strike you, and is to me, quite literal. They honestly do believe that prayer will be effective and is part of her healing process. Literally, not in any metaphorical sense. They experience these rules and restrictions as you, the staff, forcing them to neglect their mom. That is truly hard for them.

I have encountered these sorts of families before; this family is a paradigm of the matriarchal, religious, mystical family. I realize that they are more than difficult. They are so intense as to be overwhelming, . . . no question. But they are the "real stuff." . . . They do believe that their prayers and ministrations are part of the cure, part of the solution.

The plan that we forged is not perfect—indeed it may not work at all—but it was a plan that we felt would let them demonstrate good faith and let you give a bit—on the issue of weekend visiting and on the matter of the father's visits. It has all of the marks of mediation in that neither side is really happy. The nurses were not happy at least and the family is not. But, they want so much to try to remedy the mess, as do the nursing staff, with the exception of one nurse who is so mad that nothing short of tar and feathers will satisfy her. . . .

I am trying to sell this plan and give it a chance. Would I be able to do this if I were you? I am not sure. But I do know that you guys are in it together for the long haul and this might, just might, start things again. Of course not start from a clean slate, . . . that is not possible. . . . But perhaps this agreement will cool things down.

Interesting to note that Mr. Dominick was key to accepting this plan. He said "do it" and get this rolling again. The deal breaker or clincher, however, was a different rule for the husband. That became the symbolic center for their not losing face. One of the nurses said that he never stays very long in any event—of course in the perverse universe of mediation this will change immediately.

So, those are my 5 a.m. thoughts.

I sure hope that this cooling off period works—as I said I don't have great hopes but I still do harbor a few.

Dr. Kibbe arrived the next morning and agreed to the terms.

By Tuesday morning tempers had soared on both sides of the white coat rack. A meeting with the staff revealed that the family had not abided by the rules, had not called each time before entering the unit, and had not limited their visits to ten minutes. The family was equally adamant that the experiment had been a failure. Mrs. Cotrelli, Mr. and Mrs. Dominick, the two mediators, and an outside expert met in an empty room. Mrs. Cotrelli stated that she was sorry that she had agreed;

it was ridiculous that they were not permitted to visit for as long as desired, and because they were not there to say prayers, her mother had deteriorated over the weekend. Mr. Dominick stated that they would agree to no limitation of their visits and that if there were interference with their access they would soon see the hospital in court. They stated flatly that they would agree to no rules and there would be no compromise.

Because of the explosive nature of the case and the complex dynamics, Mr. Purdure and Ms. Lieland had invited an experienced mediator and teacher of mediation practice to accompany them to the meeting. He was introduced at the outset and his role explained. The participants were asked whether they had any objection to his presence and they stated no, they did not care who was or was not there. The expert was asked to comment but offered no suggestions for a resolution.

Ms. Lieland closed the discussion and stated that she and Mr. Purdure would document the breakdown of the negotiations in the chart. The visiting mediator stated privately that in order to forge a consensus and reach an agreement each side needs the same desire to reach a common point. Without that shared commitment to search for consensus the process will certainly fail; this discussion, he stated, was an example of that principle.

The mediators wrote the following note in the chart:

> We consulted on this patient last week. Because of problems with the family (interfering with the care of the patient and intimidating the staff) we were asked to become involved. We met with family and staff and all agreed to the plan. See note of last Thursday.
>
> Today we met again, according to the agreement, with staff and family. Family said at the outset that they would accept no restrictions but for a limit from 12 a.m. to 6:30 a.m. Staff at first wanted to extend 10 minutes/hour to 20 minutes/hour. Finally, we got staff to agree to unrestricted visiting from 11 a.m. to 8 p.m. with 2 limits.
>
> 1.  Family members must intercom before entering.
> 2.  Family members must leave when any nurse arrives to care for the patient.
>
> Family has rejected this and is very intimidating and threatening.
>
> We have alerted the hospital medical director who first referred the case, the risk-manager, the director of patient services, and the director of security.
>
> This attempt at mediation has failed.
>
> The family does not understand why the staff perceives them as disruptive. They absolutely reject limitations and see their presence as necessary to their mother's spiritual and emotional well-being. They are a devoted and loving family that can't understand how disruptive their behavior is.

This is a very sad case: devoted family and very caring staff who have tried to work it out. The family is now adamant and will not accept any limitation of visiting.

Common ground requires both sides to want to reach an agreement. The family sees that the policy the staff wants is not what they want—a sorry state—but no compromise possible.

One last point. The family feels that these restricted hours are making their father's health worse—he feels the pressure to be there more.

We have reported to Dr. Kibbe on the lack of an agreement and have alerted administrators.

Two days later Dr. Kibbe saw the husband in the patient's room. Despite the fact that the family had stated that Mr. Leonari should not be involved in decisions about his wife's care and only Mr. Dominick should decide about arrangements, Dr. Kibbe had continued to speak with the husband about the patient's status, new developments, and the changing prognosis. He asked Mr. Leonari before each meeting whether he wanted to be involved in discussions and he consistently said yes.

On day two after the breakdown of the negotiations, Dr. Kibbe presented the agreement to Mr. Leonari and asked him whether he thought that it was fair to the family and to the patient. He said yes, it was fair and that he would like the atmosphere between the family and staff to be better, adding that he would tell his family to abide by the rules.

The staff agreed to unlimited visiting from 10:00 a.m. to 8:00 p.m. All others agreed.

On visiting the SICU some time later, Ms. Lieland asked a visitor, a daughter she had never met, how the relationships were between family and staff. "Oh," she stated, "I don't get involved in any of that."

Two weeks later, Dr. Lordson reported that tension was beginning to mount again and asked that one of the mediators pay a visit. On arrival a day later, Ms. Lieland found that all was calm. The patient had experienced a dramatic improvement and Mrs. Cotrelli and Mrs. Dominick were tremendously pleased. Dr. Kibbe had discovered a hidden source of infection that, when drained, led to an immediate improvement in mental status, responsiveness, and kidney function. The pushing for extended hours had ended abruptly and all agreed to ask, one day in advance, for variation of the usual procedure.

Despite the efforts of an accomplished staff and a devoted family, the patient died.

## Analysis

Medicine interacts with people's lives on the planes of suffering, reliance, trust, and fear. Depending on individual wisdom, the strength of family support, one's sense of afterlife, and the effectiveness and compassion of care providers, the hospital experience can be tolerable or horrible for all involved. When conflict surrounds the process, it can magnify the negative aspects of the experience for all of the participants—family, patient, and staff—and intensify the contrasting perspectives and interests.

Mrs. Leonari's case is the story of a mediation that failed. But ultimately the compromise that had almost been forged was the plan that was implemented—so maybe it is actually the story of a mediation effort that succeeded. That effort began when the mediators started the process of communication that let the staff and the family work together or at least bump more productively against each other. It continued when they shuttled back and forth between the family and the staff, arguing alternately for the position of one or the other of the parties and suggesting the various compromises that became the basis for the new understandings and, finally, for the solution. All along the way, the mediators absorbed the anger of the family when the first attempt at forging a new plan had failed. Perhaps that is one of the chief lessons from this case and one of the salient characteristics of the hospital mediative process—the process, its intermediate steps, and its interim solutions are key components of the product.

### *Letting the Staff Express Their Feelings*

The mediators began by providing a safe space, in front of an audience who were neutral to the extent that they were unknown to the family and unfamiliar with the conflict, where the staff could come together and express their anger and frustration at the behaviors of the family. An interesting point is that some of the staff at this first meeting defended the family and tried to calm the waters and soothe the most agitated staff, especially the one nurse who had recently been reported to her supervisor. Many of the staff subscribed to the explanation of one of the surgeons that this was a loving, close, and interlocked family who had never tried to function outside of the supervision and support of the matriarch.

Midway into the discussion one of the mediators raised what is a standard bioethics analysis in the context of intensive care units. She suggested that the staff of an intensive care unit is itself a scarce resource and that the behavior of a family that seeks too much attention and therefore takes more than its proportionate share of the staff's time is not only a staff organization issue but also an issue of the allocation of scarce resources. One of the nursing supervisors pointed out that this line of reasoning, although salient, would be counterproductive for this family and actually quite explosive. The family's response was likely to be, "How you take care of your other patients is not for us to say; if our mom needs this much care, it is your responsibility to provide it."

### Helping the Family Understand the Situation

Once discussions with the family had begun and the family was confronted by the anger of the staff, they understood that a united staff, not just one or two disaffected persons, was appealing to them to change. The reality that emerged from the collective discussion of the care team could no longer be denied.

The first family members the mediator spoke with were the patient's two older daughters, who were the most evident at the SICU and who had, despite the frequent admonitions of the staff, continued to use their cell phones while in the patient's room. The mediators' task then was twofold: they must try to understand the perceptions and feelings of the family and try to convey to them the feelings and perceptions of the staff. This second part was particularly difficult because the two women emphasized again and again that their quarrel was only with one nurse. The mediators tempered their comments about the staff as a united front by repeating the compliments and praise that the staff had offered in support of this family and in recognition of their devotion to their mother.

### Identifying the Conflict as a Conflict

The most important product of this first discussion with the daughters was their agreement that there was a problem and their assertion that they would like help in solving it. With difficulty they accepted the notion that the staff shared a common perception. They did not want a fractured relationship with the staff because they realized that this tension could not be helpful to their mother's care.

Most mediators are contacted once the parties have reached an impasse and have recognized their need for help. In this case, as in all hospital settings, underscoring the existence of a conflict is an initial task for the mediators. The fact that the family wants "everything done," for example, and the staff thinks that aggressive care is not in the best interest of the patient—a common conflict—is identified as a disagreement to be solved only when the mediators enter the picture. Hospital staff and most family members are frightened by the notion of conflict and shy away from its identification. This first step, identifying conflict, is critical in that it permits both sides to see that a common plan is a necessary precondition to caring comfortably and adequately for the patient. The mediators must help both sides to see that the "best interest" of the patient can be served only by a plan that encompasses the perspectives of the care providers and the family, as well as an objective evaluation of the needs of the patient.

This case was unusual in that the conflict was not about the care provided; it was about the behavior of the family. The perception, however, that the family was intimidating the staff and interfering with the best care for the patient was as powerful a conflict as are the more usual disagreements about the care plan.

### Developing Options

Patients and family members are particularly vulnerable in the hospital setting. They are totally dependent on the staff to care for the patient, interpret the data that indicate the patient's progress or regression, advocate for the patient in the strange world of tests and consultants, and, most important, prevent death or, in the case of the very ill or terminally ill patient, permit it. The staff seem to stand in a position of unparalleled power, leaving many families reluctant to express uncertainty, discontent, anger, or frustration; all behaviors are fraught with danger. Family members fear retaliation and worry that patient care will be compromised if the staff have any negative feelings about their behavior.

The mediators are related to but separate from the staff that are actually caring for the patient. Thus, family members perceive the mediators as safer recipients for criticism, worries, and feelings of discontent. The mediators can reassure family members that their anxieties are normal and that any concerns they express, as long as they do not bear directly on the patient's condition, will remain confidential. They can serve as interpreters between family and staff, setting the framework for discussion and creating a protected space where both sides can comfortably express any emotions that might interfere with care of the patient.

### Meeting with Family and Staff

Once the mediators understand some of the issues on both sides, they try to move the sides as quickly as possible to a common understanding about the future care plan for the patient. But whereas caucusing in standard mediation might mean asking one of the sides to step out of the room to allow the mediators to have a brief discussion with the other side, caucusing in the hospital setting is a very different and far more complex matter. Just reaching all staff can require many hours because of the 24-hour nature of care, changing staff shifts, and the hierarchy of authority among staff. In this case, the mediation effort began at 2:00 p.m.; by 8:00 p.m., the mediators had spoken with most of the staff and once with the two daughters alone and again with the two daughters and the son-in-law. But since Dr. Kibbe was out of the hospital at the time the second meeting with the family took place, Ms. Lieland had to resort to the early morning e-mail message. The mediators had presented the staff's concern to the family but had not had time to reflect the family's perspective to the surgeon who, in the hierarchy, made the ultimate decision.

A second important characteristic of the caucuses in bioethics mediation is the mediators' totally transparent stance. Maintaining this stance is difficult for the mediators, however, because they have not been chosen by the family and they are employed by the hospital. And although the mediators always acknowledge this lack of independence, which Mrs. Leonari's family noted, it makes them subject to suspicions that are not normally part of the mediation process. But their position also gives them access to the staff, hospital records, hospital discussions, and staff relationships, none of which would be available to an outsider. This is, as noted below, a difficult trade-off made necessary by the setting and the stakes.

In Mrs. Leonari's case, the mediators' transparent stance is illustrated in the e-mail message to Dr. Kibbe in which Ms. Lieland acknowledges that she is trying to "sell" the solution that emerged the evening before. But the mediators were equally open with the family, promising to try to explain the position of the family to the staff but acknowledging, too, that they were also trying to "sell" the family on the need to compromise to make life bearable with the staff.

In her e-mail message, Ms. Lieland notes that none of the participants is "really happy" with the proposal. Whether everyone leaves a mediation "happy" about the outcome is not relevant; it is more appropriate to frame the goal of mediation as finding an agreement that satisfies as many of the parties' interests as possible and provides a solution all can live with.

### Being the Advocate for the Forged Solution

Once a compromise is reached, the mediator's job is to be its advocate to ensure that it is implemented. The essence of a mediated solution is the consensus about the core of the agreement. In this case the core of the agreement was the idea that the family would abide by rules and that the staff would expand the usual visiting hours.

The family followed the advice of Mr. Dominick and agreed to the restriction but then regretted the decision. The core of reciprocity held, just barely, over the test time of a long weekend. By the end of that time both sides were angry and the process was almost back to the start but for the important facts that conflict was acknowledged, each side understood more about the feelings and perspectives of the other, and a temporary solution had been proposed. Thus, the parties could never return to the state they had been in before the process was initiated. Each possessed more information and therefore a more sophisticated level of understanding than had existed before.

### Recognizing Impasse

Once it was clear that the family was not only uncooperative but also actively hostile and threatening, it fell to the mediators to call an end to their process. In any mediation both sides must want to reach an agreement before the process can succeed. If either side withdraws from good faith participation in the mediation—from openness to reaching a shared solution—then the mediation must end and other processes and forums, such as arbitration or civil court, must be sought to resolve the conflict. In Mrs. Leonari's case, once the daughters had asserted that they would not compromise, the mediators alerted the administration of the hospital that the family had withdrawn from the process and had threatened to sue. At this point the behaviors and conflicts in the case passed from the hands of the mediators to the hands of the administration, especially the medical director of the hospital and the director of risk management. The former is ultimately responsible for the care of patients and the latter for assessing the risks for possible future hospital and individual liability.

Because the family also threatened to ignore all restrictions and be present whenever they chose, not just at the times stipulated by the staff, and because the staff insisted that this behavior would not be permitted, the director of security was also alerted. In one more attempt at transparent mediative behavior, the mediators told the family that they would be required to alert the hospital administrators; once they did, they reported the fact to the family. They also informed the family that the director of security had been briefed on the matter.

The family representatives were in a rage and not inclined to listen, certainly not to compromise. Emotions were high, and they had become aggressive, seemingly more concerned with winning than with reaching a positive outcome for the mother's care. What they had not calculated on was the hospital's closing ranks and, ultimately, the father's taking a more conciliatory stance.

### Finding a Solution

Mr. Leonari's sensitivity to the needs of the staff and his ongoing connection with the surgeon director of the SICU permitted the discussion to continue and a plan to be implemented.

Despite the fact that the two daughters had stated that all communication should be with them and Mr. Dominick, the surgeon continued to talk with Mr. Leonari. He thought that this was the appropriate thing to do and was not intimidated by the daughters and the son-in-law. His line of discussion with Mr. Leonari was a lifeline for the agreement. Once Mr. Leonari learned from the surgeon about the disagreement and the structure of the solution that had been mediated, he accepted the solution and accepted the responsibility to impose it on his family.

# IV

## ROLE PLAYS: PRACTICING MEDIATION SKILLS

*The four role plays in this part have been used in the Certificate Program in Bioethics and Medical Humanities. The first two, "Discharge Planning for a Dying Patient" (Chapter 9) and "An At-Risk Pregnancy" (Chapter 10), were created in 1993 for the original project on mediating bioethical disputes by Leonard Marcus, David Matz, Jane Honoroff, and Nancy Dubler. They have evolved over the years to the form presented here. The last two role plays, "HIV and Postsurgical Complications in the ICU" (Chapter 11) and "Treating the Dying Adolescent" (Chapter 12), were developed by Linda Farber Post and Jeffrey Blustein of the Division of Bioethics as teaching tools for the Certificate Program.*

*These role plays are based on a combination of experience and imagination. They are designed to expose the peculiar challenges and configurations of bioethics mediation, including the multiplicity of players, the variability of motives, and the complexity of management. Neither this set of role plays nor any text can provide all of the skills that a mediator in bioethics consultations needs—this book is only a beginning. Bioethics consultation has a mediative and a consultative aspect. For expertise in bioethics, there is no substitute for education about the principles and normative rules that form the intellectual foundation for the practice of bioethics. For expertise in mediation, further training will also be needed.*

*This part may be especially useful for mediators working with bioethics students and professionals. It can be a self-help guide for experienced bioethics consultants who desire a new lens on practice. It can also provide the basis for workshops and classes.*

### Using the Role Plays

*Each role play provides general instructions and a list of participants (the number required varies from four to eight), and confidential instructions for each player. The player assigned the mediator role will play himself or herself as a mediator. All other parties to the mediation will be given a fictitious name. Ideally, each participant will be assigned to a role different from his or her real-life position, with the exception that at least one of the role-play doctors should be a real-life nurse or doctor or someone else with medical knowledge. Taking on a different role is important because the experience gives the role player insights into the perspectives of others in the health care system. And the experience of watching a participant take on a different role allows those who hold the roles in real life to see what assumptions about their roles others bring to role playing.*

*The four role plays are provided in order of increasing difficulty. Allow 60 to 90 minutes for each role play, including at least 30 minutes of feedback. If possible, give out the role play assignments so the participants can prepare ahead of time. When this is not possible, add 15 minutes to the time allotted for each simulation. Explain to the role players that they should work in real time. That is, they should get as far as they can in the allotted time and not try to rush even if they do not have time to complete the mediation.*

*All of the role plays use solo mediators, but we encourage trainers to adapt the solo role to co-mediators. Co-mediation increases the chance that all information will be heard and all interests identified; it also increases the likelihood that the parties will find someone across the table with whom they feel comfortable. For training purposes, co-mediation allows more participants to practice in the role of mediator. There are drawbacks, however, to which trainers should be alert; for example, some pairs may be a poor match because one mediator dominates, allowing a more tentative mediator to stay uninvolved.*

## Giving Feedback

*Begin the session by reminding the role players that the purpose of the simulations is to give trainees the opportunity to practice mediation skills. Thus, while good acting is valued, caution the parties not to get so deeply into a role that they speak at length (leaving little time for the mediators to intervene) or fail to respond to appropriate mediator moves. Also tell the mediators that during the simulation they can call time out and ask for help. Discuss with them whether they would like you to call a time out if you see them struggling during the simulation.*

*The role plays are where most of the real learning takes place. While each trainer has his or her own way of providing feedback, we recommend the following approach:*

- *Be aware of the time allotted for each role play and the division of your time with the group between role play and feedback.*

- *Take process notes—a rough running transcript with evaluative notes in the margin. These can be as simple as +, –, discuss.*
- *Plan to* spend at least a third of the allocated time *giving feedback. If the simulation is going well, you can save feedback until the end, but because of the complexity of the bioethics situations, it is likely that some intervention will be required.*
- *One intervention technique for getting the "mediators" back on track without stopping the session is for you to move behind them, temporarily take on the role of mediator by making a comment or suggestion, let the parties respond, and then return to your seat.*
- *Begin the final feedback session by asking the mediators how they thought the role play went. One advantage of this technique is that participants may be more comfortable, and thus less defensive, making negative comments about their own performances than hearing negative comments from an observer. Also, allowing the mediators to speak first lets you know immediately how much insight they have into their own performance. If the mediators accurately describe areas of difficulty, it is important that you praise them for their insight and, equally important, let them know that you agree.*
- *After getting the mediators' perceptions about how the session went, you may want to turn to the other participants for their critiques. This is a good chance for them to practice using neutral, nonjudgmental language. Sometimes, especially early in a training, trainees may be overly protective of their peers. An effective technique for dealing with this reluctance to criticize is to ask the participant to pick something he or she would have handled differently and explain it.*
- *Begin the discussion of the trainees' critiques by asking questions. To the mediators or other trainees: "How did you feel when —— said —— ?" To the mediators: "When you said/did ——, what where you thinking/feeling/trying to achieve?" To the mediators: "What would you like to have said instead?" (After this question, go into role playing with you playing the appropriate party so the mediator can practice.) These kinds of question are great teaching devices in general and are especially valuable when you run into a defensive trainee.*
- *During a feedback session, it is helpful to be descriptive rather than evaluative: "Carl, it is important for the parties to have time to take in the opening statement. If you slow down it will be easier for them to catch everything." And it is helpful to be specific. Say, "Jody, after you asked Mr. Jones what he wanted from mediation, you waited a split second and then went right on to say, 'Is it money, an apology . . . '" rather than, "Jody, you seem to have trouble tolerating silence."*

- *It is as important to give positive feedback, with lots of stroking, as it is to point out problem areas. Many people learn better from hearing what went well than from hearing what was wrong.*
- *Anything that seems troublesome or bogs your group down is probably worth sharing with the whole class.*
- *Some struggling is acceptable, but if the mediators seem to be totally lost, call for a time out. You might also simply suggest that they should wrap up the session and take a break. Then you can help during the recess.*

*Chapters 13 and 14 are annotated transcripts of simulated bioethics mediations based on the role plays "An At-Risk Pregnancy" and "HIV and Post-Surgical Complications in the ICU," respectively. These are not "model" mediations but rather examples of two mediators at work, doing their best to choose interventions that will help the participants find a resolution to the wrenching situations that led to the bioethics mediation. After participating in each role play, participants may find it helpful to read the appropriate transcript and discuss how their experience differed from the recorded one.*

# 9

## Discharge Planning for a Dying Patient: A Role Play

### General Instructions

All players should read the general instructions. Before beginning, teachers should review "Using the Role Plays," p. 135.

#### Parties

R. Klein, social worker

C. Ware, nurse

Dr. J. Hathaway, attending physician

Bioethics mediator

#### Background

Harold Hadoni is a 76-year-old colon cancer patient who is anxious to leave Perpetual Memorial Hospital (PMH). Mr. Hadoni had a bowel resection with a colostomy. The cancer has now metastasized to his liver and his spine, causing some bladder compromise. He requires heavy nursing care, an I.V., and strong pain medication. Mr. Hadoni's condition is terminal and he wants to die at home.

The question of releasing him from the hospital has become a matter of dispute among staff on Five West of PMH. Dr. J. Hathaway, Mr. Hadoni's physician at PMH, feels that, although Mr. Hadoni might derive some marginal benefit from continued medical care, there is nothing more that can be done for him in the acute care hospital. Moreover, Dr. Hathaway sympathizes with Mr. Hadoni's wish to die at home and therefore has issued an order for his discharge. But Nurse C. Ware, head nurse on Five West, believes that it is medically irresponsible to discharge Mr. Hadoni, given what is known about his medical status and his home circumstances. Mr. Hadoni, a widower, lives alone in a secluded area of the county accessible only by a dirt road. He has become estranged from much of his family, except for a 23-year-old granddaughter who lives in the large city of Beaconville, 150 miles away.

Mr. Hadoni has caught wind of the dispute and has declared that, as a World War II veteran, he will take nothing less than an "honorable discharge" to his own home on his own conditions. Mr. Hadoni insists that under no circumstances will he die in the hospital or in a nursing home. He says he is grateful for all that has been done for him in PMH but that now it is time to get ready to say good-bye. He wants to spend his remaining time in a place that is familiar and comfortable—in the wild, with his trees, his animals, and his memories.

Dr. Hathaway is a well-respected physician. Active in a number of local medical society committees, he/she believes that, while medicine's first responsibility is to the patient, the profession also has a moral and social responsibility to help control health care costs. The best way to do this is to use the appropriate level of care for each patient. Hospitals should be used only when required by the patient's acute condition. Since he/she has gone public with this sentiment, he/she believes he/she must follow it in the way he/she renders care. To do any less would be to compromise his/her credibility. Moreover, Dr. Hathaway is under pressure to discharge this patient. Mr. Hadoni's managed care medical insurance policy limits the length of his hospital stay and his number of covered days has almost run out.

Nurse Ware has a different view of this case and the role of hospitals in general. He/She is a 40-year veteran of hospital nursing and has seen trends come and go. But the one principle that has not changed for him/her has been the highest concern for the welfare of the patient. He/She has seen the obsession among health care providers and hospital administrators with early discharge grow over the past ten years, causing havoc for many patients and their families. This obsession also has had the unintended side effect of making his/her job more difficult, because the patients who remain in the hospital are far sicker and require more care. Certainly, most patients can manage with a quick discharge. But over the years, Nurse Ware has seen many instances where the interests of the patient have been sacrificed to the concerns of social and administrative efficiency.

The case of Mr. Hadoni, Nurse Ware believes, is typical of this trend. A man this sick and with this little support should not be sent home. Although the possibility of nursing home placement has been raised, Mr. Hadoni is unwilling to sign the papers that would authorize his discharge to a nursing home. Indeed, it is not even clear that a nursing home could handle his care. And, to Nurse Ware's dismay, Dr. Hathaway, knowing all that, still wants to send him home.

R. Klein, one year out of his/her master's degree program at the State College of Social Work, joined the staff of Five West as a social worker just three months ago. In that time, he/she has found that much of the work at PMH, for which his/her degree work did not prepare him/her, boils down to discharge planning: working with the staff, working with the patient and family, and connecting them to local services. Klein has found that since PMH is not located in a large metropolis like Beaconville, there are few services available in the area. Furthermore, the belief persists among many patients and families that if you are sick, you belong in the hospital.

Klein's boss, the director of the Department of Social Services, made it clear when Klein was hired that the job of the social worker at PMH is to move the patient out of the hospital as efficiently as possible. A record of continual efficient discharges has been responsible for the increased respect and recognition that the department has received.

Klein has done some investigating about Mr. Hadoni's case and has some good ideas for solutions. Unfortunately, his discharge has become such a contentious issue between Dr. Hathaway and Nurse Ware that neither has shown any interest in sitting down and looking at the options. Dr. Hathaway said, "Nursing home or discharge to home" in the last conversation, emphasizing that there was no need or time for further discussion. Nurse Ware said, "No way," emphasizing too that there was no need for further discussion.

### The Request for Mediation

The social worker, R. Klein, frustrated with the impasse, has called the Bioethics Committee to request a consult. A member of the Bioethics Committee has been asked to mediate a meeting of Dr. Hathaway, Nurse Ware, and Klein to see whether there might be some resolution to the case.

## Confidential Player Instructions

### Discharge Planning for a Dying Patient
*Bioethics Simulation*
*Confidential Instructions for* **R. KLEIN,** *social worker*
*(Please do not show these instructions to the other parties.)*

You never scored high on those assertiveness tests. You are particularly intimidated by well-known doctors such as Hathaway or hard-crusted nurses like Ware. But in this case, you think you have developed some workable options. Although you have tried to raise your questions to both Dr. Hathaway and Nurse Ware and even to explain what you've learned in your research, you have found both of them to be more concerned with their principles than they are with the patient.

The information you have uncovered may provide the basis for resolution of the conflict. You know that Mr. Hadoni has a granddaughter and he has told you that they have a very close relationship. She seems to be the only person in the family who has been able to connect with him. However, she is a student at a local college, where she is now completing her exams. She has been working her way through school, and graduating with good grades has been important to her and her grandfather. In fact, Mr. Hadoni has forbidden her to come to the hospital until she has finished her exams, two days from now. Although he never had much money, he has contributed what he can to help her through school. He often reminds her that his dream has been to see her hold a college diploma, the first ever in the family. She is a pre-med student and over the years has spent many hours doing volunteer work in hospitals. She has cared for her grandfather in the past and may be able to stay with him over the summer, but you are not certain whether these plans are firm.

You are not sure whether there is a Visiting Nurse Association (VNA) in that part of the county. Nurse Ware would know more about that. There is also mention in the medical record of a local physician, but you know nothing about him or his availability.

You have had several interviews with Mr. Hadoni. He seems at peace with his terminal condition and he knows what is ahead of him. He has been an independent man and proud of having been in control all his life. He told you that he wants to do the same thing with death that he did with life.

You believe that a discharge plan that meets everyone's concerns can be developed. The question is whether Dr. Hathaway and Nurse Ware are interested in putting one together.

***Discharge Planning for a Dying Patient***
*Bioethics Simulation*
*Confidential Instructions for* **DR. J. HATHAWAY,** *attending physician*
*(Please do not show these instructions to the other parties.)*

If you had to spend this much time and energy debating every hospital discharge, you would have virtually no time to practice medicine. Between the social worker and the nurse, they should have been able to figure some way to move this case along.

You have seen plenty of patients like Mr. Hadoni; his is precisely the type of case for which physicians rightly get so much heat. If, indeed, Mr. Hadoni can benefit from further medical care, there are nursing homes that can care for him just as well as PMH can and for far less money. If he does not want to go to the nursing home, the social worker should sit down with him and persuade him to sign the papers. More to the point, you argue that he is in possession of all his faculties and, if he still insists on going home, he should be allowed to do so. That is his right. This is not a medical problem. This is a social problem and hospitals are not social service agencies.

You want to see this problem over and done with in not more than 24 hours! One day is far more than necessary to resolve a matter as simple as this. You are feeling pressure from all sides. Mr. Hadoni's insurance coverage is about to run out and you do not want the hospital stuck for further days while people try to make discharge decisions. You have kept your average length of stay admirably below that of other physicians at PMH and you want to keep it that way.

If Mr. Hadoni is insistent about going home, you do know a doctor, Edward Sylvan, out in his part of the county. You met Dr. Sylvan at a medical society meeting and he mentioned that he is willing to do home visits for his patients as long as there is good Visiting Nurse Association (VNA) back-up. Sylvan's name appeared in the medical chart, so some home support arrangement might be possible.

Because this has become such a complex and far-reaching case, you are concerned that it will set a precedent for similar cases in the future. You are concerned about patient well-being but equally concerned about cost containment. Someone has to make the hard decisions. It would take some strong persuading for you to change your mind.

*Discharge Planning for a Dying Patient*
*Bioethics Simulation*
*Confidential Instructions for C. WARE, nurse*
*(Please do not show these instructions to the other parties.)*

The hospital is facing the prospect of a large liability suit if Mr. Hadoni is discharged. Moreover, releasing a man as ill as Mr. Hadoni is unethical. If Dr. Hathaway wants to become president of the state medical society, the campaign should not be waged on the backs of the patients at PMH. His/Her outspoken support for controlling medical costs and patronizing admonishments of medical colleagues for not joining the effort have alienated many doctors and nurses, even beyond the walls of PMH. It's time to put an end to this unprofessional and unethical behavior.

It is true that there are patients in Mr. Hadoni's condition who have received adequate post-hospital care in a nursing home. But this case is different. Mr. Hadoni has confided to you that his wife died in a nursing home. He said to you just two days ago, "Mark my words, I would commit suicide before I go into one of those places." You are convinced that he was not kidding.

And his delusions about life at home must be seen in their proper context. You have never been out to his part of the county, but you do know that there cannot be much out there short of trees and bears. He may *think* he knows what is in his best interest, but sending him back there would be irresponsible. He told you about his loving 23-year-old granddaughter who is ready to take care of him. But this is probably just another delusion as well. In all the time he has been here at PMH, she has not visited even once. His own daughter was here twice and, in both instances, relations seemed strained. He probably cannot depend on her for help.

You do know that there may be some services available in the section of the county where Mr. Hadoni lives. You have heard about another patient near Mr. Hadoni's home who is receiving intensive Visiting Nurse Association (VNA) care. But it is not clear that the VNA could handle someone in Mr. Hadoni's condition. The nurse assigned to the area would have to have some of her responsibilities reassigned. It would take at least three days to arrange it, and maybe more.

You are willing to listen, but there is a point to be made in this case that cannot be compromised. Hospitals were built to take care of patients, even patients like Mr. Hadoni. You do not care what some bureaucrat says at the managed care headquarters, or what Dr. Hathaway says here at PMH. It would take some strong convincing for you to change your mind.

*Discharge Planning for a Dying Patient*
*Bioethics Simulation*
*Confidential Instructions for **BIOETHICS MEDIATOR***
*(Please do not show these instructions to the other parties.)*

This is a difficult situation compounded by the fact that you have some tough characters around the table. The issue is more than one of medical ethics alone. There are clashes of personality, as well as significant social, professional, and managerial issues at stake. Everyone seems to have a strong position to defend.

You need to find a resolution that addresses all of the issues in this case. Otherwise, problems will fester and may well come up with other patients.

You may not reach a final decision in this case today. However, you do want to establish the criteria for eventually making a decision, including determining what facts, information, or conditions will trigger a decision for each option. If these particulars can be established, the case can be moved along without the need to reconvene this group.

You are concerned that one or all of the parties may leave the negotiating table before a resolution is achieved. The legitimacy of the Bioethics Committee is still questionable at PMH and, you realize, at the table here as well.

# 10

## An At-Risk Pregnancy: A Role Play

### General Instructions

All players should read the general instructions. Before beginning, teachers should review "Using the Role Plays," p. 135.

#### Parties

Hans Olsen, patient's husband          Dr. Leah Prince, obstetrician
Dr. Ron Walker, obstetrics chief resident          Bioethics mediator

#### Background

Southend General Hospital is a busy urban hospital. Its ambulatory care center serves the many low-income residents who have no other resource in the area. Thanks to a generous long-term grant from the federal government, it has a busy maternal and child health clinic (MCHC) that provides a comprehensive set of services, allowing it to care for women through their pregnancy and into motherhood.

A problem has arisen in the care of one of the regular patients of the MCHC. A 32-year-old woman, Cindy Olsen, is in her 18th week of pregnancy. She and her husband, Hans, have one child, a six-year-old girl. There have been three recent miscarriages. Mrs. Olsen has been extremely apprehensive about her pregnancy, worrying and constantly asking questions about her diet, her husband's work environment, and her medical care. The medical team working with Mrs. Olsen agrees that her anxieties are excessive, even for a woman with so many miscarriages.

On an ultrasound of the fetus, Mrs. Olsen's obstetrician, Dr. Leah Prince, notes that the structure of the fetus's heart does not seem quite right. She has her suspicions, but she is not sure whether there is really a problem or whether the appearance of an anomalous heart is caused by the angle at which the ultrasound was taken. Dr. Prince wants to repeat the ultrasound and do a fetal echocardiogram to rule out a heart defect. A confirmed defect in the structure of the heart could be very bad not only because the heart problem might be quite serious but also because the defect could indicate some chromosomal abnormality.

Dr. Prince has been seeing Mrs. Olsen and her husband for the past seven years, from the birth of their first child through all the miscarriages. They have developed a very warm professional relationship. Dr. Prince, a mother, and a doctor for 31 years, believes that sharing her findings and their possible implications with Mrs. Olsen at this point would cause Mrs. Olsen extreme distress. If Dr. Prince's suspicions are not confirmed, she reasons, she will have spared Mrs. Olsen needless suffering. If her suspicions are confirmed, she will have time later on to discuss the implications of her findings with Mrs. Olsen and her husband.

The obstetrics chief resident, Dr. Ron Walker, has been involved with Mrs. Olsen from the start of this pregnancy. Dr. Walker is upset because he feels that it is inconceivable that a doctor would withhold information about the first ultrasound from the parents. Such a move would deny Mrs. Olsen the right to full information about her baby and the right to decide about her own health and that of her child.

### The Request for Mediation

Dr. Prince has decided to call for a medical ethics consult to help resolve the question of whether or not to tell Mrs. Olsen about the doctors' concerns. (The patient, Mrs. Olsen, is not an active role-player in this exercise. This simulation goes to the point where a decision is made about whether to tell her, how to tell her, and what to tell her.)

## Confidential Player Instructions

*An At-Risk Pregnancy*
*Bioethics Simulation*
*Confidential Instructions for **HANS OLSEN**, patient's husband*
*(Please do not show these instructions to the other parties.)*

Cindy's intense anxiety weighs heavily on you. Indeed, you worry yourself that all her tension cannot be good for her health or that of the baby. Still, she has come through three miscarriages pretty well psychologically, and you believe that deep down she is a strong woman. You are reinforced in this belief after talking with Cindy's close friend Carol. Carol and Cindy have had long talks about the pregnancy, and Carol—a very level-headed person—continues to reassure you.

The real cost of all the tension around the pregnancy is the strain on your marriage. Cindy never misses a chance to worry about the microwave (that you bought), your halogen lamp, your computer screen, the carbon monoxide from your car, and even—once—the garlic on your breath from lunch. You have tried to humor her. But you have also exploded, with increasing frequency lately, because she has seemed almost to enjoy and need these worries.

Your biggest hope is that the pregnancy will go smoothly and produce a healthy child, and then the relationship will revert to its usual assumptions of sharing and trust. Another miscarriage will be tough for Cindy, and for you. It might also force the decision to consider pursuing adoption, something both of you have resisted until now.

You trust Dr. Prince, and as long as Cindy is well cared for and gets what she wants, you will be satisfied.

*An At-Risk Pregnancy*
*Bioethics Simulation*
*Confidential Instructions for* **DR. RON WALKER**
*(Please do not show these instructions to the other parties.)*

You have finally exposed Dr. Prince as the rigid, power-hungry tyrant she is. She sometimes pretends to a little feminist chic, but really she cares only that doctors make all the decisions, and by that she really means doctors with centuries of experience, not residents.

There could hardly be a clearer case for a patient's autonomy. Who else should decide about the welfare of a fetus if not the mother? Dr. Prince is wildly exaggerating—as she often does—about the potential harm to the mother and fetus from telling about the possibility of a heart defect. But even if she is accurate in her prediction, who appointed her God? Even the risk management people would agree that Mrs. Olsen has to be told. The last thing the hospital needs is a lawsuit because a patient failed to get crucial information.

Of course, if the decision is made to tell Mrs. Olsen and it results in causing her harm, that might put you on the spot as the advocate for informing her. That would give Dr. Prince all the ammunition she would ever need in future battles with you. It would be awfully nice to find a way out of this corner.

You are not happy about the possible impact on your career of being in conflict with a senior physician, but all in all, this is a matter of principle. You went into medicine because of your commitment to certain values. Informing the patient about her condition is one of those values.

*An At-Risk Pregnancy*
*Bioethics Simulation*
*Confidential Instructions for* **DR. LEAH PRINCE,** *obstetrician*
*(Please do not show these instructions to the other parties.)*

You are troubled by this case for several reasons. First, there is the danger to the patient. Second, there is a matter of precedent that concerns you. From your point of view, Dr. Walker is more concerned about patients' rights than about patients. Yes, there is a place for the principle of informing patients about their condition. But each patient is different, and each piece of information is different. If the individual needs of each patient are ignored in the name of some higher principle, then we have done a great disservice to patient care. This is an example of the ideology of patients' rights run wild.

You are quite sure that the resident assigned to you, a young man, is chortling over the position that this case puts you in. He becomes the champion of a woman's right to decide and you appear as an antifeminist. He has more than once made clear his dissatisfaction with your view that a doctor's first, and often only, responsibility is to the patient's physical well-being. He has chided you for being simplistic whenever this topic has come up. He has, for example, accused you of ignoring other interests, including patient autonomy and the psychological welfare of patients. The two of you have never discussed the matter in depth. Your position in this case just reinforces the image you know the younger house staff have of you as a rigid old traditionalist. You think this image is unfair and inaccurate.

You would like to get out of this corner. If you do not tell Mrs. Olsen about the ultrasound and she finds out later that you had suspicions you did not share with her, she may be very angry with you. You also have to find some way to deal with the echocardiogram. You truly like the Olsens and do not want them to despise you, much less to sue you.

This is a tough one. But as the physician for the Olsens for all these years, you believe the decision is yours.

### An At-Risk Pregnancy
*Bioethics Simulation*
*Confidential Instructions for* **BIOETHICS MEDIATOR**
*(Please do not show these instructions to the other parties.)*

You have served as the on-site medical ethicist at Southend General Hospital for six years. It has been a fascinating, though taxing job for you. Several hours ago, you received the call from Dr. Prince. This latest case from the MCHC seems to be another real challenge.

As a first step you called the Office of Risk Management. The director of Risk Management told you that telling Mrs. Olsen is definitely the safer route from a legal point of view. The results of the ultrasound must be included in the medical record. Those records could be used as evidence later if the Olsens decide to take legal action.

You take the view that all the relevant parties need to work together, and that your task is to bring about that collaboration. While you hope Dr. Prince and Dr. Walker will be able to resolve their differences, you are not required to bring them to the same conclusion. Your role is to give each a full chance to hear and explore the views of the other so that the outcome can be greater clarity about their own and others' motives and the alternatives, as well as an agreement or a more sophisticated set of alternatives to choose from.

Your preliminary hypothesis about the case is that the key question is whether to tell Mrs. Olsen, how to tell Mrs. Olsen, and what to tell Mrs. Olsen.

As in any group process, there needs to be a decision about whom you should involve in these discussions. Then you must decide how to begin. Do you bring all the relevant players together for an opening conversation or meet with them one at a time or in subgroups? These choices are yours.

# 11

## HIV and Postsurgical Complications in the ICU: A Role Play

### General Instructions

All players should read the general instructions. Before beginning, teachers should review "Using the Role Plays," p. 135. Assume that this mediation occurs in New York.[1]

### Parties

Mr. and Mrs. Abruzzi, patient's parents

Dr. A. Schwartz, immunologist

Dr. B. Heinstein, oncologist

T. Chen, social worker

M. Aquino, ICU nurse

J. Henry, risk manager

Bioethics mediator

### Background

Frankie Abruzzi is a 37-year-old man, currently in the intensive care unit (ICU). He admits to IV drug abuse in the past but claims he stopped using drugs several years ago. Seven years ago Frankie tested positive for HIV, and five years ago he was started on AZT. Also significant in his medical history is a heart valve replacement several years ago due to endocarditis (inflammation of the tissue surrounding the heart) contracted through his drug use. According to his parents and immunologist, Dr. A. Schwartz, who has known Frankie for several years, Frankie has coped fairly well emotionally with his condition and has been very conscientious about taking care of himself. Recently, Frankie was divorced from his wife. He has tried to maintain contact with his young daughter.

In August, Frankie was referred by Dr. Schwartz to Dr. Heinstein, an oncologist, because of an elevated white blood cell count. A bone marrow biopsy was done, and

---

1. In New York and Missouri, a decision to stop treatment must be based on the patient's prior expressed preferences.

Frankie was diagnosed with a very early stage of CML, a form of leukemia. Interferon was started six weeks later but was discontinued shortly thereafter because Frankie continued to spike fevers. According to Dr. Heinstein, Frankie's leukemia is definitely treatable.

While in the hospital, Frankie developed abdominal swelling due to fluid buildup. He also developed an acute retroperitoneal bleed, for which he was transferred to the ICU. The bleeding was coming from his right kidney, which was removed one week ago. Postsurgery, Frankie has not recovered consciousness. He is on a ventilator, and so far weaning attempts have proved unsuccessful. He also has low blood pressure and has developed renal failure, for which he has received dialysis on three occasions. Unfortunately, because of Frankie's low blood pressure, dialysis has had to be discontinued, at least temporarily. There is no health care proxy for the patient and no living will.

Frankie's parents seem genuinely concerned about doing what is best for Frankie and sparing him any unnecessary suffering. The day dialysis was started, Frankie's parents walked into his ICU room and were shocked to see yet more tubes and machines hooked up to him. They asked for a do not resuscitate (DNR) order. The surgical resident provided one and Mrs. Abruzzi signed it. The social worker, T. Chen, witnessed the signing. The parents also told Dr. Heinstein, who was Frankie's attending physician at the time, that they wanted dialysis stopped and no further aggressive treatment instituted. Dr. Heinstein explained to the family that he/she could not agree with their decision about resuscitation, dialysis, and other treatments. In his/her view, the patient's condition was potentially reversible, that is, the patient might be "salvageable." Dr. Heinstein stated that he/she does not want to continue to be Frankie's physician under these circumstances. Dr. Burrows, the renal attending, stated that though Frankie is critically ill, if his blood pressure can be raised it would make sense to resume dialysis. If it cannot, then the issue of dialysis might be moot.

### The Request for Mediation

At this point, M..Aquino, a staff nurse in the ICU, called the bioethics mediator. The mediator set up discussions with two of the doctors involved with the case, Dr. Heinstein and Dr. Schwartz. Dr. Burrows was out of town at a conference and could not attend.

**Confidential Player Instructions**

*HIV and Postsurgical Complications in the ICU*
*Bioethics Simulation*
*Confidential Instructions for* **MR. ABRUZZI,** *patient's father*
*(Please do not show these instructions to the other parties.)*

You are unsure about what is best for Frankie, though your wife feels very strongly that aggressive treatment should be stopped. Since you are somewhat intimidated by your wife, you did not strenuously object to her signing the DNR order. You have been pressing the physicians for a clear prognosis and do not know how optimistic to be. But you do know that Frankie has always been a fighter and that he's a person who loves life, and so you are pretty certain that Frankie would want everything done for him now and would not want to forgo care. During the meeting, you disagree, somewhat hesitantly, with your wife about termination of care. If you are comfortable with the way the meeting is going and if you receive adequate information and emotional support, you may agree to have the DNR order revoked and dialysis resumed when appropriate.

*HIV and Postsurgical Complications in the ICU*
*Bioethics Simulation*
*Confidential Instructions for* **MRS. ABRUZZI,** *patient's mother*
*(Please do not show these instructions to the other parties.)*

Your greatest concern is that Frankie not suffer. Because Frankie occasionally pulls at his tubes and grimaces, you are afraid that he is in pain and you want the treatment causing it to stop. You continually press the physicians to talk to you about Frankie's prognosis. What really is his chance of returning to any kind of normal life? Even if Frankie should get over his postoperative complications—which you feel is extremely unlikely—he will still face a future with AIDS.

You feel very strongly that aggressive treatment should be stopped. You believe that Frankie's prognosis is grim and he is in pain and suffering for no good purpose. Your husband is less sure than you are about termination of treatment and you have argued with him about it. Also, you had to persuade your husband to agree that you should sign the DNR order. If you are comfortable with the way the meeting goes and receive adequate information about management of Frankie's pain, as well as emotional support, you may agree to revoke the DNR order and resume dialysis if and when it becomes possible.

*HIV and Postsurgical Complications in the ICU*
*Bioethics Simulation*
*Confidential Instructions for* **DR. A. SCHWARTZ,** *immunologist*
*(Please do not show these instructions to the other parties.)*

You do not feel as strongly as Dr. Heinstein does about the inappropriateness of a DNR order or stopping aggressive treatment. You believe that Frankie is critically ill and may very well not recover to leave the hospital. Should he arrest, resuscitation may very well be medically futile. Even if it is not futile, resuscitation would likely impose an extraordinary burden on Frankie in the light of his medical condition and the expected outcome of resuscitation. You are less sure about the appropriateness of discontinuing dialysis.

In terms of pain management, you believe that Frankie is being adequately sedated. In general, you are not adamant that it is morally appropriate to sign a DNR order and withdraw aggressive treatment. You are willing to concede, however, that under the circumstances, Mrs. Abruzzi's position wanting the DNR is not unreasonable.

*HIV and Postsurgical Complications in the ICU*
*Bioethics Simulation*
*Confidential Instructions for* **DR. B. HEINSTEIN,** *oncologist*
*(Please do not show these instructions to the other parties.)*

You do not agree with the DNR order or with Mr. and Mrs. Abruzzi's wishes to stop all aggressive treatment for Frankie. The CML is in an early stage and treatable with chemotherapy. Frankie may be weanable, his peritoneal bleeding has stopped, his ascites is being treated, and his mental status may improve. Furthermore, there is no way of knowing how much longer Frankie can live with HIV. He has already made it seven years. Finally, resuscitation would not be futile or necessarily extraordinarily burdensome. You believe that the HIV issue must be separated from post-op issues so that the HIV issue does not unduly influence people's thinking about what is appropriate care for Frankie. In your view, the situation is not hopeless. You may want to remind the mediator and Dr. Schwartz that the renal attending, Dr. Burrows, agrees with you that additional treatment is appropriate.

You believe strongly that it is morally wrong not to treat Frankie aggressively and morally wrong to enter a DNR order. You are not conciliatory and you are convinced of the moral correctness of your position. You see it as your obligation to do everything you can to help Frankie as long as there is a possibility of improvement.

*HIV and Postsurgical Complications in the ICU*
*Bioethics Simulation*
*Confidential Instructions for* **T. CHEN,** *social worker*
*(Please do not show these instructions to the other parties.)*

When you witnessed Mr. Abruzzi's signature on the DNR order, you thought the family fully understood Frankie's condition and prognosis. You believe that Frankie is critically ill and that his parents are within their rights to consent to a DNR order and request termination of aggressive treatment. The family, in your view, has a great deal of moral decision-making authority in such cases. You are aware that, under New York State law, their ability to make termination-of-care decisions is strictly limited. You (incorrectly) believe that since the family may sign a DNR order, the right to authorize termination of care goes with it. You believe that withdrawal of life support is quite appropriate in Frankie's case. But you are confused about what your role should be in the mediation. What should you do about the DNR order?

*HIV and Postsurgical Complications in the ICU*
*Bioethics Simulation*
*Confidential Instructions for* **M. AQUINO,** *ICU nurse*
*(Please do not show these instructions to the other parties.)*

You take pride in the care you provide Frankie and do your best to comfort his parents as they wrestle with this wrenching decision. You see your job as offering emotional support to Frankie's family. When you suggested to the family that it might be helpful to speak with a bioethicist, you did not make it clear to them that the bioethics consultation is advisory only and that the ultimate decisions about Frankie's care belong to his attending physician.

*HIV and Postsurgical Complications in the ICU*
*Bioethics Simulation*
*Confidential Instructions for J. HENRY, risk manager*
*(Please do not show these instructions to the other parties.)*

You are concerned first about the hospital's liability, not necessarily what is best for Frankie. As legal adviser to the hospital you are able to describe the legal situation in New York State regarding DNRs and withdrawal of life-sustaining care. There are four medical predicates—terminal condition, persistent vegetative state or PVS (irreversible severe neurological damage, leaving the patient unaware of his or her surroundings and unable to recognize and relate to family and friends), medical futility, and extraordinary burden—at least one of which must be satisfied before anyone but a health care proxy can consent to a DNR order for an incapacitated patient. Stopping dialysis, an issue that may come up in the mediation, requires either a health care proxy or clear and convincing evidence of the patient's prior wishes in this matter. The clear and convincing evidence standard is very demanding. General information about the patient's values is not sufficient. The evidence must relate specifically to the patient's condition and must show a firm and settled conviction to refuse aggressive treatment under these circumstances. Since there is neither a proxy nor clear and conclusive evidence from a legal point of view in this case, your stand is that withdrawal of dialysis is out of the question.

*HIV and Postsurgical Complications in the ICU*
*Bioethics Simulation*
*Confidential Instructions for BIOETHICS MEDIATOR*
*(Please do not show these instructions to the other parties.)*

Your working hypothesis going into the mediation is that the following issues will be discussed:

1. patient's current condition
2. patient's prognosis
3. family's understanding of these issues
4. family's wishes regarding continued aggressive treatment
5. patient's previously expressed wishes, if any; patient's values, outlook on life

During the meeting, you may have to decide whether to point out that the goal of medicine is not simply to provide all available treatment but to provide the treatment that is medically and ethically appropriate. You might mention that there is a significant bioethics literature arguing that withdrawal of dialysis may sometimes be ethically appropriate. And you might also discuss the importance of trying to determine the patient's wishes regarding treatment and what is in his best interest.

# 12

## Treating the Dying Adolescent:
## A Role Play

### General Instructions

All players should read the general instructions. Before beginning, teachers should review "Using the Role Plays," p. 135.

### Parties

Mr. and Mrs. Ajuba, patient's parents        L. Harper, risk manager
Dr. K. Salazar, oncologist        Bioethics mediator
H. Albright, social worker

### Background

Lucy is a 17-year-old Kenyan female who was diagnosed with cancer 18 months ago. At the time of diagnosis, the cancer had invaded one kidney and metastasized to bones, lungs, liver, and aorta; Lucy's prognosis was fairly poor given the extent of the metastases. Lucy underwent surgery to remove the diseased kidney six months prior to this hospitalization. She began a nonexperimental course of chemotherapy, but she showed no improvement. She was therefore placed on an experimental chemotherapy protocol. A scan done two months ago showed new metastases in her shoulders and bones. By the time of her admission, Lucy was experiencing significant abdominal pain, most of which could be controlled through the use of an analgesic patch.

Shortly after her admission her pain problems increased, and Lucy was admitted to the Pediatric Intensive Care Unit (PICU) in renal failure. She continued to experience significant pain, which was again controlled with an analgesic patch. During her stay in the PICU, she was often very restless and unable to lie still even though every movement was painful. She was also terrified because she was clearly getting worse instead of better. In addition, her abdomen had become quite distended. She repeatedly asked why her "belly" was "so big." After a few days in the

PICU, she was stabilized and transferred back to the ward, but her remaining kidney was, in the words of her oncologist, "a disaster."

Lucy is emotionally immature for her age and unusually dependent on her parents, especially her mother. Both of Lucy's parents have been involved in her care from the beginning. They are both very religious and have repeatedly expressed their faith that God will cure their child. They lost their only other child to malaria before they moved to the United States. Her father has described Lucy's illness as a "white man's disease." From the time of diagnosis to the present, both of Lucy's parents have insisted that she be told nothing about her prognosis or her medical status. Nonetheless, Lucy has given some indications that she is aware that her disease is serious and, more recently, that she is terminally ill. Throughout the course of her illness, Lucy's father has insisted that she receive all possible treatment to keep her alive. Lucy's mother has not opposed her husband's orders but is generally more accepting of her daughter's condition and prognosis.

Shortly after Lucy was transferred out of the PICU, her oncologist, Dr. K. Salazar, stated that a do not resuscitate (DNR) order would be appropriate, that her tumors needed to be reevaluated, and that it was probably inappropriate to continue curative treatment. He/She therefore raised the subject with Lucy's parents. After considerable reluctance, the parents agreed to the order. The following day, however, the parents rescinded the order, and there was some indication that Lucy's father had pressured his wife into this action.

Now, a few days later, significant changes have begun to occur in Lucy's condition. It has deteriorated and worsened to the point that she has had to be readmitted to the PICU and intubated. In the PICU she has continued to deteriorate, and within the past 24 hours she has experienced four episodes in which her blood pressure has fallen to a dangerously low point, each of which was treated aggressively. She is receiving escalating support to maintain respiration, blood pressure, and other vital signs. In addition, her level of pain and discomfort requires heavy sedation.

### The Request for Mediation

The treating team, including physicians, nurses, and social workers, is concerned about the appropriateness of continuing aggressive curative treatment. Lucy's oncologist has sought a bioethics consultation to discuss appropriate treatment. A meeting has been set up to discuss the ethical issues in the case.

## Confidential Player Instructions

*Treating the Dying Adolescent*
*Bioethics Simulation*
*Confidential Instructions for **MR. AJUBA,** patient's father*
*(Please do not show these instructions to the other parties.)*

Your faith is strong. You believe that God will save Lucy and that it is the responsibility of the hospital to keep her alive until God does his work. You are adamant that everything possible be done for your daughter. You see Lucy's cancer as "a white man's disease" that she never would have contracted if you had not brought your family to the United States. For that reason you sometimes blame yourself for her illness. Despite Dr. Salazar's recommendation, you believe very strongly that Lucy's sedation should be reduced or eliminated in the PICU so she can regain full consciousness. Your wife pressured you into signing the DNR order. When demanding that the DNR order be revoked, you said to your wife, "If Lucy dies it will be on your head."

### Treating the Dying Adolescent
*Bioethics Simulation*
*Confidential Instructions for* **MRS. AJUBA,** *patient's mother*
*(Please do not show these instructions to the other parties.)*

You do not want to continue living if Lucy dies. You believe Lucy's physicians about her prognosis and you want to follow their recommendations. In your culture, family harmony is valued and a wife defers to her husband, so it is difficult for you to challenge your husband's insistence on continued aggressive care for Lucy. You think your husband feels responsible for Lucy's illness: if he had not brought the family to the United States, Lucy would not be dying of this "white man's illness." You reluctantly agreed to sign the DNR order. When your husband then demanded that the order be rescinded, he said to you, "If Lucy dies it will be on your head."

*Treating the Dying Adolescent*
*Bioethics Simulation*
*Confidential Instructions for* **DR. K. SALAZAR,** *oncologist*
*(Please do not show these instructions to the other parties.)*

In your medical judgment, Lucy's prognosis is hopeless. With aggressive treatment, Lucy may be able to get through her current crisis, but all she has to look forward to is a few more months of physical and emotional suffering. You now advocate that Lucy's level of treatment be scaled back and that the goal be provision of palliative care, even if this results in her death, as is probable. You have been frustrated in your efforts to deal with Lucy's parents. Mr. Ajuba does not seem able to hear these facts, and Mrs. Ajuba appears too emotionally fragile to handle this forecast.

Up to this point, you have acceded to the wishes of Lucy's parents regarding both aggressive treatment and not communicating to Lucy the gravity of her condition. But now you are deeply conflicted, torn between not causing Lucy further suffering and honoring her parents' instructions out of a sense of moral obligation, as well as fear of their wrath. You feel strongly that Lucy should be kept sedated in the PICU because without sedation she would experience a great deal of pain both from her disease and from the ventilator tube in her throat. You are thus distressed by Mr. Ajuba's demand that Lucy be permitted to regain consciousness. You believe that if Lucy were to recover to the point of breathing on her own, it would be more difficult to keep her pain free and impossible to keep her both pain free and conscious.

You also are deeply disturbed about the fact that Lucy has never been informed about her condition and has never had the opportunity to participate in decision making, even though she has given indications of her ability to do so. You regret not having taken a more forceful stand on this issue earlier.

## Treating the Dying Adolescent
*Bioethics Simulation*
*Confidential Instructions for* **H. ALBRIGHT,** *social worker*
*(Please do not show these instructions to the other parties.)*

You appear to be the only person in whom Lucy has confided her awareness of her condition and her fears of dying. Lucy told you that she does not want her "heart to stop" and that she does not want to be alone when she "gets sicker." She also indicated on several occasions that she was thinking about and afraid of dying, especially dying alone.

You have felt very uncomfortable about not being able to discuss with Lucy the likelihood and the circumstances of her dying. However, you believe that as long as the medical staff are acceding to the parents' wishes not to disclose this information to Lucy, you must also accede.

You have talked with Mr. and Mrs. Ajuba about cultural norms and familial bonds. They told you that since Lucy is their only remaining child, her death would mean the end of the family line, and this possibility is deeply upsetting to them.

***Treating the Dying Adolescent***
*Bioethics Simulation*
*Confidential Instructions for **L. HARPER,** risk manager*
*(Please do not show these instructions to the other parties.)*

Your first responsibility is to protect the hospital from liability. You do not agree with Dr. Salazar's recommendation that Lucy's level of care be scaled back to focus on palliation. You are worried that the hospital is "walking into a lawsuit." Going against the parents' wishes for life-sustaining treatment for their child is potentially legally explosive and puts the hospital at unnecessary risk. You feel that the parents will be less angry and more accepting if Lucy's death is delayed, giving them more time to adjust to the inevitable and reassuring them that everything possible has been done for their child.

*Treating the Dying Adolescent*
*Bioethics Simulation*
*Confidential Instructions for* **BIOETHICS MEDIATOR**
*(Please do not show these instructions to the other parties.)*

You have been consulted by Dr. Salazar at a time of extreme turmoil among the health care team and the family. There are strong feelings on the part of the care-givers that the goals of care for Lucy need to be revised in her best interest. Great distress is evident over the unwillingness of the parents to recognize the validity of the medical judgments and the inevitability of the suffering Lucy will experience with continued life-sustaining treatment. You are disturbed that the issue of communicating with Lucy was never squarely addressed by the caregiving team, and you feel this issue should be raised during the mediation. Another issue that must be resolved is that of Lucy's sedation and pain control. Your working hypothesis going into the mediation is that you will need to lead a discussion about Lucy's current condition and prognosis, her family's understanding of the condition and prognosis, family and provider wishes regarding treatment, and Lucy's previous and potential for future involvement in her own care and decision making. You hope the mediation will result in a plan of care that respects the wishes and feelings of the parents as far as this is possible, without compromising the well-being of their daughter. It is also necessary to recognize and support the professional integrity of the caregivers. A central issue in the mediation is what constitutes "unacceptable suffering."

# V

## ANNOTATED TRANSCRIPTS OF BIOETHICS MEDIATION ROLE PLAYS

*The two chapters that follow are annotated transcripts of simulated mediations that were conducted during the 1999 spring semester retreat for the Certificate Program in Bioethics and Medical Humanities. They have been slightly edited for teaching purposes. The commentary added throughout the transcripts calls the reader's attention to the use of mediation skills. The mediator for the at-risk pregnancy role play (Chapter 13) was one of the students in the course. The mediator for the HIV role play (Chapter 14) was a professional bioethics mediator.*

# 13

## An At-Risk Pregnancy:
## A Role Play Transcript

### Background

A 32-year-old woman, Cindy Olsen, is in her 18th week of pregnancy. She and her husband, Hans, have one child, a six-year-old girl. There have been three recent miscarriages. Mrs. Olsen has been apprehensive about her pregnancy, worrying and constantly asking questions about her diet, her husband's work environment, and her medical care. The medical team working with Mrs. Olsen agrees that her anxieties are excessive, even for a woman with so many miscarriages.

On an ultrasound of the fetus, Mrs. Olsen's obstetrician, Dr. Leah Prince, notes that the structure of the fetus's heart does not seem quite right. She has her suspicions, but she is not sure whether there is really a problem or whether the appearance of a heart anomaly has been caused only by the angle at which the ultrasound was taken. Dr. Prince wants to repeat the ultrasound and do a fetal echocardiogram to rule out a heart defect. A confirmed defect in the structure of the heart could be very bad for the baby not only because the heart problem itself might be quite serious but also because the defect could indicate a chromosomal abnormality.

Dr. Prince has been seeing Mrs. Olsen and her husband for the past seven years, from the birth of their first child through all the miscarriages. They have developed a warm professional relationship. Dr. Prince, a mother, and a doctor for 31 years, believes that sharing her findings and their possible implications with Mrs. Olsen at this point would cause Mrs. Olsen extreme distress. If Dr. Prince's suspicions are not confirmed, she reasons, she will have spared Mrs. Olsen needless suffering. If her suspicions are confirmed, she will have time later to discuss the implications of her findings with Mrs. Olsen and her husband.

The obstetrics chief resident, Dr. Ron Walker, has been involved with Mrs. Olsen from the start of this pregnancy. Dr. Walker is upset because he feels that it is inconceivable that a doctor would withhold information about the first ultrasound from the parents. Such a move would deny Mrs. Olsen the right to full information about her baby and the right to decide about her own health and that of her child.

Dr. Prince has called for a bioethics consult to help resolve the question of whether or not to tell Mrs. Olsen about the doctors' concerns.

## Annotated Transcript

*Doctors Prince and Walker meet with the bioethics mediator.*

**Bioethics mediator:** All right. Well, I think, Dr. Prince, you know me. I know you know Dr. Walker. Dr. Walker, I'm the medical ethicist at Southend General Hospital, and I've been here for six years. Dr. Prince has called me in so that we can talk about what to do about Cindy Olsen. And I've called in the two of you to speak alone initially. What I'd like to do is to get the two of you to explore what are the medical limitations for Cindy Olsen: what are the possibilities, what are our roles in taking care of her. And, ultimately, what's the best course of action for her, if she should be told, what she should be told; and if she is told, what kind of support she might need. So, I think, Dr. Prince, you've known Mrs. Olsen for the longest, so I wonder if you'd start by telling us a little bit about her history and her condition.

> *The mediator starts with introductions. She reframes the issues to focus on the patient's needs rather than on the disagreement between the doctors and maintains that frame as she asks Dr. Prince to speak. By starting with Dr. Prince, she chooses to defer to the hospital hierarchy. This approach seems appropriate here as a way both to get information about the patient care issues and to build trust with Dr. Prince, who is under attack by the resident. In other situations the mediator might find it useful to go against the existing power structure and start the conversation by having someone lower in the hierarchy speak, thus sending the message that during the mediation everyone's views are important and will be heard.*
>
> *The mediator's use of the words "called in" ("Dr. Prince has called me in," and "I've called in the two of you") could cause a misunderstanding. In lay terms those words have a bit of a scolding tone. In medical settings consults may be "called in" to give an opinion in a case. Using that language in mediation may set up an expectation that the mediator will be presenting an option or making the decision.*

**Dr. Prince:** I've been Cindy's obstetrician for seven years. She has one child who's six. Subsequent to that, she had three miscarriages. She's now at the 18th week of her pregnancy. She had an ultrasound last week, which revealed an abnormality—what appeared to be an abnormality in her baby's heart. I don't know if it's a function of bad positioning of the machine, or whether it really reflects an abnormality. What I would like—the other thing I'd like to mention is that Cindy's a very anxious, overly nervous person, patient—everybody agrees that she's excessively nervous, even though she's had three miscarriages. What I would like to do is have this ultrasound repeated to clarify the evidence as to whether there is a heart abnormality or not. And I'd also like to get an echocardiogram. However, given Cindy's history of anxiety, I don't want to tell her what I'm doing or, let us say, I don't want to tell her that I think there may be a heart abnormality in the fetus. I would just like to tell her the films didn't come out, or the pictures didn't come out, and I'd like to repeat it. That's my position. I feel that in order to protect Cindy's peace of mind it would be better to go ahead, do the tests, get the final results, get more definitive results, and then, if they reveal there's a problem, talk to her about them.

*Bioethics mediator:* OK. Well, the husband does not know at the present time?

*The mediator asks a quick clarifying question.*

*Dr. Prince:* Neither the patient nor the husband.

*Bioethics mediator:* Dr. Walker, tell us about your contact with Cindy—what your feelings are about that?

*This is an open-ended question for Dr. Walker.*

*Dr. Walker:* Well, I'm the chief resident, and I've been with her since the beginning of the pregnancy. I'm aware of all of the situations leading up to this point. The ultrasounds we've done have not confirmed a heart defect at this point. My problem right now is realizing that the patient does not have the information that we have. And so I'm very concerned about concealing, which is exactly what we're doing, concealing important information that the patient has a right to know.

*Dr. Prince:* My feeling is that by informing her you're just going to exacerbate her mental state, which is precarious at the moment. And nothing is lost by telling her that we just need to repeat the test. Then we'll get a more definitive result, and then we'll tell her. We've lost nothing but a week, or even a couple of days.

*Dr. Walker:* Some things that come up for me, some issues are the fact that I do know this patient, and she tends to be quite anxious. She's hyper-alert to any signs of problems. If she, I believe, feels that we are doing additional tests, she's going to have anxiety far beyond anxiety that she may get if we give her a reasonable explanation. You bring a patient like this in for their procedure, another ultrasound—we would be misleading her, actually, lying to her, if we told her the films didn't come out. If you tell her that you're going to do an echocardiogram, that's further indication to a patient like this that there are other problems. And I think you're going to end up in the same anxious state, perhaps an even worse one, but you will have violated a patient's right to know her condition, and you'll lose trust.

*Bioethics mediator:* Let me clarify some things, if I can. You both think that she's an anxious patient. Would you explain a little bit about what she's done that's led you to believe that this is going to be anxiety producing?

*The mediator is transparent about what she is doing, saying, "Let me clarify some things." She highlights an area of basic agreement between the doctors: that they are dealing with an anxious patient. She then asks a narrower, but still fairly open, question, seeking information.*

*Dr. Prince:* Well, she's constantly questioning the medical instructions I give her, asking questions about her diet, about her well-being, whether her husband's job had anything to do with the prior miscarriages. Just much more so than any other—than most patients I have and, certainly, much more than her first pregnancy.

*Bioethics mediator:* Has she done anything that's unusual? Can you describe a little more of what she does? How does this affect her life, or her family?

*The mediator asks further clarifying questions. Asking multiple questions allows the respondent to talk about whatever is most comfortable. One drawback, however, is that the respondent may choose the questions that allow him or her to avoid talking about difficult subjects that need to be discussed.*

*Dr. Prince:* I'm not aware of any particular action she's taken, I just—you know, it's a practical matter. I think, living—having a wife and mother in such a state of high anxiety has got to be difficult for the other members of the family.

*Bioethics mediator:* Has the husband expressed this to you?

*Dr. Prince:* No.

*Bioethics mediator:* Have you spoken to him about it?

*Dr. Prince:* No.

*Bioethics mediator:* OK. And could you give us some information about the miscarriages?

*The mediator slips into a fact-finding mode here, asking for information that is unlikely to help resolve this dispute.*

*Dr. Prince:* She's had three prior miscarriages. They've been fairly recently.

*Bioethics mediator:* And has this—

*Dr. Prince:* Not that I'm aware of.

*Bioethics mediator:* Have you both seen the ultrasound that shows a possible heart defect?

*The mediator is back on track, asking for information that will help problem solve. Here she makes sure that both doctors have seen the critical test result, that they are operating with the same information. This question begins a series of narrow questions by the mediator.*

*Dr. Walker:* I have seen it.

*Dr. Prince:* Yes.

*Bioethics mediator:* And, you said that this was going to be a matter of days.

*Dr. Prince:* Yes.

*Dr. Walker:* Yes. Assuming that we get her in for an ultrasound fairly quickly.

*Bioethics mediator:* OK. After the repeat ultrasound and cardiogram are done, do you feel that there's going to be a degree of certainty about what you can tell the patient?

*Dr. Prince:* More than there is now. I certainly hope we know that, obviously, the baby could keep moving, and wind up in the same place. But I think we'd have a much better fix on whether there are any heart abnormalities.

*Bioethics mediator:* But it's still possible that you might have to wait another several weeks and repeat the test again, in order to have a level of certainty that you would like to have?

*Dr. Prince:* That's possible. I hope it wouldn't happen.

*Bioethics mediator:* Dr. Walker—well, maybe both of you could address this. It seems that, in the best scenario, there would be an issue of several days involved before this test is done. Dr. Walker, what is the importance of these few days to you?

*The mediator invites Dr. Walker, who has not spoken much, to become active in the conversation.*

*Dr. Walker:* I have a tremendous concern, if this turned out to be very bad news for the patient and she needed to consider an abortion, that she would be running out of time. I don't know that she's thinking this, but I, as her doctor on her case, I'm trying to look at this from the patient's perspective. And this is why I'm adamant about the patient's need to know. This is of utmost importance to her, and for her family, and for the future of this child. And I think it is unethical not to tell her.

*Bioethics mediator:* Will her knowledge about a possible heart defect be crucial?

*Dr. Walker:* I believe it will be.

*Bioethics mediator:* So then, going ahead with the testing has to precede her making any decision?

*With this and the previous question, the mediator is moving the focus of the doctors away from a debate about principle and toward the practical aspects of the situation.*

*Dr. Prince:* But she has a lot of time. She's only in her 18th week of pregnancy. She has until the end of the second trimester, which is another—I understand the risk increases as the weeks go on, but she's got time. She's not in the 27th week.

*Dr. Walker:* But even if that wasn't the outcome, the fact is that we have information about this patient which is very critical, and we are keeping it from her. And I believe the ethics of our situation demands that we share this information with this patient. There is no clinical reason for us to withhold information.

*Dr. Prince:* There is a clinical reason. She is highly anxious, and I'm afraid that—if the information were 100 percent certain, I wouldn't have a problem. But as it is now, we're uncertain about the clarity of the films, and we have a patient who might be adversely affected, just by the simple fact of telling her this and then making her wait.

*Dr. Walker:* However, that's hypothetical. We don't know. We don't know whether the fetus has a heart defect and we also don't know that the patient is going to become anxious. This is staff's impression of the patient. She's done nothing to evidence her anxiety.

*Dr. Prince:* Well, I've known this patient for seven years.

*Dr. Walker:* She hasn't been—

*Dr. Prince:* She's really—I know this patient much better than you do. You've only seen her for six months.

*Dr. Walker:* But the present time is when I'm seeing her now. The past seven years may have been that way. And, in fact, in the past seven years, you haven't been able to mention one time that her anxiety has put her in jeopardy.

*Dr. Prince:* Well, there's physical jeopardy, and then there's mental jeopardy. Increasing a person's level of anxiety is jeopardy.

*Dr. Walker:* We have no psychiatric liaison, information as to the fact that the patient is overly anxious, and it's damaging her present—

*Dr. Prince:* But we all agree that she's excessively anxious, even for a person who's suffered three recent miscarriages.

*Dr. Walker:* I wonder if it's not staff anxiety that we're talking about. We're talking about reports from the staff. We don't hear from the husband.

*The mediator has allowed the exchange between the doctors to go on until it es-calates and then intervenes with another clarifying question.*

**Bioethics mediator:** Let me just ask you again. You've felt that it was very impor-tant to report this information to the patient as soon as it's received by the staff.

*At this point it would have been helpful to summarize before asking the question. For example, "Let me take a minute to summarize where I think we are now. You both agree that Cindy Olsen is an anxious patient, though you may differ about what should follow from that fact. And you both have seen the ultrasound and agree that the results are inconclusive but that it shows a possible cardiac defect, and that if there is a defect, the patient needs to know about it so she and her hus-band can make some hard choices. And it sounds as though you both agree that the test should be repeated and that it can be done in the next few days." This sum-mary narrows the dispute by highlighting the areas of agreement.*

*The mediator might then have gone on to acknowledge the doctors' feelings and interests with statements such as: "It seems clear that both of you are committed to this patient and are concerned about her well-being and that you both have strong views about how best to care for her. Dr. Prince, you have cared for Cindy through the birth of her first child and the subsequent miscarriages and you have seen the impact of those losses on her and want to minimize the stress of this preg-nancy, and Dr. Walker, you are sensitive to Cindy's stress level, but you are con-cerned that keeping information from her now may make it harder for her in the long run and you also see this as a matter of principle about a patient's right to in-formation." The mediator, by showing that she understands both the feelings and the interests of the two doctors, may eliminate, or at least cut back on, their need to carry on their battle. Then the mediator might have gone on to break the dis-pute into more manageable pieces, saying, "And it sounds as though there are two issues we need to spend some more time on: what Cindy should be told about the reason for the repeat test and when that information should be given." Such a statement by the mediator would make the issues that need to be resolved explicit and focus the doctors on the problem that needs solving.*

**Bioethics mediator:** (For continuity, the last statement from the transcript repeats.) Let me just ask you again. You've felt that it was very important to report this information to the patient as soon as it's received by the staff.

**Dr. Walker:** Right.

**Bioethics mediator:** But that the delay of two days, so that there could be more conclusive information—

*Dr. Prince:* That's absolutely right. I think this notion that the patient has to know everything we know as soon as we know, it's not correct. I think there's room for discretion. In this case, I think discretion is warranted.

*Bioethics mediator:* Is there any decision that the patient would be taking or that she would have to take that could potentially be made in the next two days, if she were told today?

*Dr. Walker:* Well, to my way of thinking, the patient needs to be informed about these other procedures, and she would have to give an informed consent. Without the proper information, she cannot give a valid informed consent about an echocardiogram and a repeat of the ultrasound.

*Dr. Walker reverts to a positional response. The mediator should note the response and consider the significance of this reversing. It is not unusual to have parties circle back to earlier stages of a mediation, especially when they are being asked to make choices.*

*Bioethics mediator:* How would you feel about involving the patient's husband in this decision? Because he is dealing with her, he may have some insights into her mental condition about this situation. How would you feel about that?

*The mediator makes a proposal. The basis for this proposal, however, is not clear. She needs first to do some information gathering about the husband, his role during his wife's treatment, and their relationship.*

*Dr. Walker:* I would be very reluctant to do that. I think it puts a terrible burden on the husband, to give him information which you then tell him he can't tell his wife. That poisons the well. I would not want to do that. I don't think that's good for Cindy.

*Bioethics mediator:* Well, don't forget, we're talking about two days.

*The mediator, having thought of the option of involving the husband, seems to be pushing it.*

*Dr. Walker:* I don't care whether it's two days or 20 minutes. I just don't think it's the right thing to do. I don't think it's morally right to ask one marriage partner to conceal this information.

*Dr. Prince:* I agree with my colleague, but for different reasons. I feel that we're talking about patient confidentiality, and that we must not go to the non-patient and give the information that the patient rightfully needs. And I don't believe time is the real issue here. I think it's the actual concealment of information.

*The doctors both reject the mediator's proposal. Note that she made the proposal as a question so it was easy for the parties to say no.*

*Dr. Prince:* I think time is absolutely the only issue. We wait 48 hours, we get more definitive information, and we—the possibility exists that we may never have to tell Cindy anything about this heart, that the baby's heart may be perfectly fine, and then the problem is gone.

*Dr. Walker:* The problem remains, because we're still concealing from the patient her condition, and the possible condition of her child.

*Dr. Prince:* But we don't know definitively what the condition is.

*Dr. Walker:* Then tell me how you're going to get an informed consent from the patient on two procedures without telling her the reason why.

*Dr. Prince:* You tell her that—

*In the previous exchanges the discussion escalates as the doctors reiterate their differing positions. Dr. Walker raises an important question but phrases it as a challenge.*

*Bioethics mediator:* This was actually going to be my next question to you and, that is to say, what would you like to tell the patient at this point, before she goes for these procedures? And how would you propose to answer her, if she starts asking you pointed questions?

*The mediator steps in and reframes the question so that it is not a challenge. Note her choice of words and the way she breaks down the problem into smaller pieces. She shifts from how Dr. Prince is going to get informed consent to what she would like to tell Cindy and how she will answer if Cindy asks pointed questions.*

*Bioethics mediator:* Tell me what you feel would be a reasonable way to approach Cindy, in terms of asking her to do these two procedures. How would you put this to her? And how would you handle the situation, if she starts to ask you pointed questions?

*The mediator clarifies further and gives Dr. Prince the opportunity to, in effect, practice her conversation with Cindy.*

*Dr. Prince:* I would approach her by saying that the ultrasound was taken at the wrong angle, and that there's an area of the baby's heart that we were unable to see clearly, and we need to repeat the procedure to do this.

*Bioethics mediator:* Would you be comfortable with that explanation?

*The mediator does a quick check with Dr. Walker.*

*Dr. Walker:* I think I would be, because it seems to deal with the facts as we know them. It isn't a distortion of facts. It represents what we have.

*Bioethics mediator:* OK. Well, suppose that she needs to go for an echocardiogram. What would you tell her then?

*The mediator returns to Dr. Prince and continues walking her through, step by step, what will happen in her conversation with Cindy. This is a form of reality testing.*

*Dr. Prince:* I would say that we've seen something on the film that is slightly abnormal, and we want to confirm it or rule it out by having an echocardiogram.

*Bioethics mediator:* Now, how will you approach Cindy, if she becomes very agitated? Do you feel that there's going to be something that you will have to tell her now?

*Further reality testing by the mediator.*

*Dr. Prince:* I don't know. I would have to play it by ear. I would not lie to her, I just wouldn't volunteer the information.

*Reality testing, asking specifically what Dr. Prince would do if Cindy asks questions, produces a response that is very different from the position Dr. Prince was taking that Cindy should be protected.*

*Bioethics mediator:* How would you feel about that?

*The mediator checks again with Dr. Walker.*

*Dr. Walker:* It's sounding a bit more reasonable. We absolutely can't keep from her anything that we definitively know. But my concern is getting her through to have these tests done, which we really need to do. But, also, to walk a fine line respecting her right to information.

*Dr. Walker, having heard that Dr. Prince does not propose to lie to Cindy, is able to acknowledge that the conversation proposed by Dr. Prince is "reasonable" but surrounds this acknowledgment with continued positional posturing. In this situation it is important that the mediator hear the agreement and let the rest of the statement go. Dr. Walker also may need time to absorb the fact that he and Dr. Prince really do not disagree when it comes to practicality rather than principle.*

*Bioethics mediator:* So, let me see if I understand this. We have two possibilities. One is that you tell Cindy that the ultrasound was taken at the wrong angle—and that she goes through with the test, and we then have definitive answers to tell her one way or the other. The other possibility would be that, in the process of explaining to Cindy, she asks specific questions which make it necessary for us to divulge our concerns at the present time. Am I understanding our options correctly? Are there other options that we have?

*The mediator, rather than jumping on the agreement, summarizes the options. By doing so she gives the doctors time to absorb the fairly significant concessions each has made.*

*Consider her use of the words "we" and "us." In the second sentence it is appropriate to say "we" since the options are the result of discussion between the mediator and the two doctors. In the third and fourth sentences the use of "we" and "us" is not appropriate, since the mediator will not be participating in those discussions.*

*Dr. Prince:* In other words, we leave it up to the patient to point out the direction she wants to go. And if she does ask very deliberate, pointed questions, we would give her more information and not hold any back.

*Dr. Walker:* We have to.

*Bioethics mediator:* Now, have we considered what the role of the husband is in this process? Is there anything that you'd like to say to the husband to help hold him back, so that he doesn't come in and ask the questions for her? Would you like to share with him just enough so that he does not ask those pointed questions?

*Note that in course of the discussion, references have become depersonalized. The doctors and the mediator have shifted from referring to the patient at least some of the time by her name, Cindy, to calling her the patient. In this intervention by the mediator, Hans Olsen is also depersonalized. He is "the husband." Just as earlier in the discussion the mediator shifted focus from the dispute between the doctors to the needs of the patient, here she should get back to that focus by using their names.*

*Dr. Prince:* Well, I suspect that we would not be able to talk to the wife without the husband present or, at least, that she would then go and talk to her husband. So I propose we tell the husband and wife the same thing. And then, if he asks pointed questions which, certainly, as a practical matter, would be near her or in front of her, we'd have to answer the questions.

*Bioethics mediator:* So, you would feel that it would not be productive to speak to her husband, take her husband aside, and express that he not ask too many questions at this point?

*The mediator is again trying to sell her idea or deal with her concern about the husband.*

*Dr. Walker:* No. For the same reason that I said earlier, that I don't think you can put that burden on one of the partners.

*Dr. Prince:* And, again, it's an ethical situation. It's confidential information for the patient. I would hope that we could tell the patient that we would like to discuss her ultrasound, and would she like to have her husband present. That way, we can deal with that confidentiality issue. Again, we can't conceal from him, or even hope that he won't ask pointed questions, because it's his right to ask whatever questions and our responsibility to answer them.

*Dr. Walker:* I agree with that.

*Bioethics mediator:* Then, as I understand it, we have agreed that you're going to try to schedule her ultrasound, with or without an echocardiogram, within the next two days. And that the patient will be told that, because of the angle of the baby, the heart couldn't be clearly seen and, for this reason, the ultrasound will have to be repeated. If the baby hasn't moved enough, then we'll do an echo to further delineate the specters of the heart. That this is necessary because, at this stage, we need to check all of these factors, and it's a routine procedure, and that, once the tests will be finished, then we can get the results.

*Dr. Prince:* Yes.

*Dr. Walker:* I agree.

*Bioethics mediator:* I want to thank both of you. It is clear you are both very committed to Mrs. Olsen and I'm glad you've been able to agree on ways to work together in taking the next step.

## Further Discussion

There are some common themes in this mediation: the desire on the part of some doctors to make decisions that are "best for the patient" without involving the patient or the patient's family, and the cultural clash between young doctors trained in an era of informed consent and more senior doctors who are comfortable with a more paternalistic approach.

One issue that was not discussed in this mediation but that the mediator needed to be aware of was the likelihood that Dr. Walker would be committing professional suicide if he could not find a way out of the confrontation with a senior attending. So an unarticulated need of Dr. Walker was to save face while backing down.

The role play (Chapter 10) was written with the husband, Hans Olsen, as one of the players. He is included to confront the mediator with two choices: whether to include him and, if so, when. This mediator made the decision not to speak with him separately from his wife. She felt that the disagreement was between the two doctors and that she should try to resolve things between them. If successful, she would not have to deal with whether to involve the husband. The mediator recognized that he was not a party at this stage in the dispute.

Even if the decision were to include the husband, in bioethics disputes when there are disagreements among members of the treatment team the better practice is for the mediator to meet first with the medical staff, either to resolve their differences or to clarify those differences and decide how they will be presented to the patient or the family.

# 14

## HIV and Postsurgical Complications in the ICU: A Role Play Transcript

### Background

Frankie Abruzzi is a 37-year-old man, currently in the intensive care unit (ICU). He admits to IV drug abuse in the past but claims he stopped using drugs several years ago. Seven years ago Frankie tested positive for HIV, and five years ago he was started on AZT. Also significant in his medical history is a heart valve replacement several years ago due to endocarditis (inflammation of the tissue surrounding the heart) contracted through his drug use.

In August, Frankie was referred by Dr. A. Schwartz to Dr. B. Heinstein, an oncologist, because of an elevated white blood cell count. A bone marrow biopsy was done, and Frankie was diagnosed with a very early stage of CML, a form of leukemia. Interferon was started six weeks later but was discontinued shortly thereafter because Frankie continued to spike fevers.

While in the hospital, Frankie developed abdominal swelling due to fluid buildup. He also developed an acute retroperitoneal bleed, for which he was transferred to the ICU. The bleeding was coming from his right kidney, which was removed one week ago. Postsurgery, Frankie has not recovered consciousness. He is on a ventilator, and so far weaning attempts have proved unsuccessful. He also has low blood pressure and has developed renal failure, for which he has received dialysis on three occasions. Unfortunately, because of Frankie's low blood pressure, dialysis has had to be discontinued, at least temporarily. There is no health care proxy for the patient and no living will.

The day dialysis was started, Frankie's parents walked into his ICU room and were shocked to see him hooked up to yet more tubes and machines. They asked for a do not resuscitate (DNR) order. The surgical resident provided one and Mrs. Abruzzi signed it. The social worker, T. Chen, witnessed the signing. The parents also told Dr. Heinstein, who was Frankie's attending physician at the time, that they wanted dialysis stopped and no further aggressive treatment instituted. Dr. Heinstein explained to the family that he could not agree with their decision about resuscitation, dialysis, and other treatments. In his view, the patient's condition was potentially reversible. Dr. Burrows, the renal attending, stated that though Frankie was critically ill, if his blood pressure could be raised it would make sense to resume dialysis. If it could not, then the issue of dialysis might be moot. At this point, a staff nurse in the ICU, M. Aquino, called the bioethics mediator.

## Annotated Transcript

*Mr. and Mrs. Abruzzi; Drs. Heinstein and Schwartz; M. Aquino, the ICU nurse; T. Chen, the social worker; and J. Henry, the risk manager, meet with the bioethics mediator.*

**Bioethics mediator:** Good morning. Thank you all for agreeing to come together this morning. I think that I have met most of the staff and I had a brief opportunity to talk to Mr. and Mrs. Abruzzi earlier today. Good morning to both of you. I especially appreciate your coming since I know something about this case and realize that this is a very difficult time for both of you.

Let me explain my role today. I am trained as a lawyer but have worked at this hospital for 25 years and have developed the program in medical ethics. In 1978 I founded the Bioethics Consultation Service, which is often asked to participate in discussions about cases in which difficult decisions need to be made. It is my task, or the job of my two colleagues in the service, to try to convene all of the parties so that everyone can hear each other. We don't come to make the decision. We come to be certain that all of the medical facts are on the table and that all of the options for action have been stated and considered. When possible, our goal is to help the patient, family, and medical staff to reach a consensus about a plan of care that all are comfortable with and that will guide the medical interventions provided. So that is why I asked you all to come together today and I thank you all.

Now, let us take a moment and have each of you introduce yourself and explain your role in Frankie's care and treatment. [Introductions omitted.] Thank you all very much.

*The mediator begins by introducing her role. Next she lets the family know that she has some information about the case and shows empathy for what they are going through. Then, after establishing her expertise, she quickly and concisely explains the goals of the session—giving the parties a chance to hear each other; getting out all the medical facts; identifying and considering options; reaching consensus if possible. Finally, she asks each participant to introduce himself or herself and ex-*

*plain his or her role. Even though Mr. and Mrs. Abruzzi probably know the team members, in any mediation, starting with introductions ensures that family members understand each staff member's role.*

**Mr. Abruzzi:** Can we talk about the DNR order now?

**Bioethics mediator:** Well, if you would not mind, I would like to put that off for just a while. One of the issues in thinking about a DNR order is what the physicians hope or expect might be the possibility of recovery. So, if we could put off the discussion for just a bit perhaps I am hoping that we will have more facts to consider and discuss together. I promise you, Mr. and Mrs. Abruzzi, that we will not end this discussion today before we have decided about the DNR order. I realize that this order seems the most important decision to be made, but let us try to understand what is happening medically with your son, first, and then consider all of the possibilities for actions, second. Is that OK? [All participants nod assent.] Good.

*The mediator responds to Mr. Abruzzi's attempt to begin the mediation with a discussion of the DNR by proposing an alternative way to structure the discussion— to focus first on obtaining medical facts. In doing so she expands the grounds on which the decision will be made. She reassures him that the DNR question will be addressed and acknowledges how important this issue is for the parents.*

**Bioethics mediator:** As I think everyone knows, Dr. Schwartz and Dr. Heinstein, you have differing opinions about what the course of Frankie's treatment should be. So, would you mind beginning, Dr. Heinstein, and telling us what you think is going on with Frankie's new diagnosis of cancer. I am sure that we all appreciate that for Frankie's family this seems to be the last straw; how could their son get any sicker? But I must admit that sometimes, as a nonphysician, I am amazed by how sick a patient can seem and how hopeful the physicians can remain. So, Dr. Heinstein, could you review the medical facts and tell us what you think is happening with Frankie.

**Dr. Heinstein:** Well, let me explain why I did not want to agree with the DNR order that the—

**Bioethics mediator:** Dr. Heinstein, let me interrupt for just one moment. If you would not mind, could we leave the discussion of the DNR order for a bit later? I promise everyone that we will get to this discussion before we break. But for now let us all try and understand what is happening with Frankie. I realize that it is a very complicated picture and difficult to sort out, but since the family is responsible for deciding about this order, I would like them to have as much information as possible before they have to grapple with this task.

And, before you return to the issues, Dr. Heinstein, may I ask you and all of the other medical staff to try to speak in terms that a nonmedical person would understand. One of my mentors once said, "Remember, the doctor speaks doctor and the nurse speaks nurse and no one speaks patient or family." So, let us return to Dr. Heinstein. Thank you for letting me add these few words—

*At the outset of any bioethics mediation, the mediator faces an important decision about who should speak first. He or she can start with the person with information, the person who initiated the consult, the person who needs to be heard, the person of higher rank, or the person of lower rank. There are no rules for making this choice, but it is important to be aware of the advantages and disadvantages of each choice.*

*Also, it is important early in the mediation to have one of the participants state the medical facts, especially where several physicians are involved in the patient's care, since the medical facts will be the basis of subsequent discussion. Often, even among health care providers involved with a specific patient, there are misconceptions about the medical facts. These facts can be clarified by having one doctor pull them all together and state them for the group. Moreover, medical facts are always in flux. Tests and monitors produce ever-changing data and doctors differ on the meaning and interpretation of the data. The mediator tries to obtain agreement on the facts before moving the discussion to the meaning that treatment team members assign to those facts and the doctors' theories about what is going on (their differential diagnoses), what treatment alternatives are available, and what is likely to happen in the future (the prognosis).*

*Beginning with a statement of the medical facts has five advantages. First, as in the opening sessions of all mediations, the initial description of the situation provides a common base on which to build future discussions. Second, it allows those who have additional information to provide it. Third, it sets the stage for clarifying questions by others at the table. For example, the social worker may have questions about the patient's condition or prognosis that he or she needs to have answered in order to develop a discharge plan. Fourth, the simple pulling together of the medical facts may make it clear that controversial treatment or discharge plans are not going to work, so that what seemed to be a serious area of disagreement simply disappears. Finally, providing a clear explication of the medical facts can sometimes eliminate the conflict, especially in situations where they have not been effectively communicated to the family.*

*In this case, the bioethics mediator chose to start with Dr. Heinstein, the oncologist, whom she saw as the source of the problem, rather than with Dr. Schwartz, who was in charge of Frankie's care and therefore in a position to give the most complete overview of the facts. The information the mediator had before the ses-*

*sion suggested that the parents wanted a DNR order but were being pressured by Dr. Heinstein to withdraw it. The bioethics mediator decided to let Dr. Heinstein speak first in order to get a sense of his current position. She entered the mediation expecting, because of her experience with oncologists, that Dr. Heinstein would be the most difficult participant in the mediation.*

*When asked, during a debriefing of this mediation, why she decided to invite the oncologist to speak first, the mediator acknowledged that her history with oncologists had made her biased. She expected that Dr. Heinstein would want to treat this patient until the moment the patient crashed. She entered the mediation with information that suggested it might be time to stop treatment, expecting to deal with a physician whose approach was that it is never time to stop treatment. No mediator can be unbiased. Each is influenced by his or her life experiences. What is critical and is demonstrated by the mediator in this case is that the mediator be aware of her bias. Here she remains open to the possibility that she is wrong; and, not withstanding the fact that she has preconceptions, she treats Dr. Heinstein impartially.*

*Other mediators might chose to start with Dr. Schwartz in order to elicit a complete overview of the medical facts, possibly in a less contentious tone. The mediator needs to take time to think through the pros and cons as he or she decides on the initial order of speakers. It is also important to remember that mediation is a very forgiving process. Usually the only cost of making a wrong judgment about the timing or order of speakers is that it will take more time to gain the trust of the participants and obtain a clear sense of the issues that need to be addressed in the mediation.*

*Beginning mediators often think they should allow the person who initiated the consult to speak first. In some cases that approach may be appropriate, but in others the initiator may have a heightened perception of conflict, which is likely to be expressed in ways that set an unnecessarily contentious initial tone. In addition, depending on where the person who initiated contact with the bioethicist fits in the hospital hierarchy, he or she may be feeling vulnerable and prefer to avoid the initial spotlight.*

*Notice that in this case the mediator does not identify the person who initiated the consult and no one asks who did so. In a well-designed program, anyone in the medical center can ask for intervention by a bioethicist. The bioethics mediator should be prepared to deal with situations where participants want to focus attention, and possibly blame, on the initiator, rather than on the problem that needs to be solved.*

*Often, part of the agenda of the mediator is to reveal who asked for the intervention in a setting where resentments about making the dispute "public" can be*

192   *Bioethics Mediation*

*dealt with. Such might be the case if a junior person calls a consult and in doing so angers the senior attending physician.*

*Early in Dr. Heinstein's presentation he (like Mr. Abruzzi) raised the issue of the DNR order. The DNR order had been the focus of a positional battle involving members of the treatment team and Frankie's parents about the proper response to Frankie's deteriorating condition. Without the mediator's intervention to postpone discussion of the DNR issue, the participants would probably have focused on positions and, while doing so, found it difficult to listen or give information. The mediator's again saying, "We'll get to that later. We're not going to do that now," allowed all parties to relax and listen rather jump to battle mode to defend their positions. At the same time she indicated her awareness that this was an issue that would need to be addressed.*

**Dr. Heinstein** (after summarizing the medical facts as set out above): So you can see that we can't hold off on the DNR decision for very long.

**Bioethics mediator:** So Dr. Heinstein, let me just understand from your perspective, you came in as the oncologist for the patient, and he has a leukemia which you think is possibly treatable. He may get better from this leukemia, but we would have to get his blood count up and get him back on dialysis, but you think he could get better?

*Dr. Heinstein responds to the bioethics mediator's deferring of the DNR discussion with a statement that could be taken as a challenge to the mediator's proposed structuring of the discussion. Rather than treating the doctor's statement as a challenge, the mediator responds by summarizing the presentation of medical facts and his assessment of the prognosis. She then checks with him to be sure she has heard correctly. This checking with the speaker also demonstrates the mediator's respect for the speaker and is an important way of validating the speaker's participation in the process.*

*At this point the bioethics mediator might also have checked with the family to see whether they had any questions about the medical facts or had learned anything new.*

**Dr. Heinstein:** Yes indeed.

**Bioethics mediator:** Dr. Schwartz, could you give us a little history of you and the patient and tell us where you think the issues are now.

*This is a fairly open question by the mediator. By asking for a history of the physician and the patient and for the physician's assessment of the issues, the mediator provides a frame that draws attention to the patient rather than to the conflict between the doctors.*

*Dr. Schwartz:* Well, I started taking care of Frankie several years ago, but transferred the care to Dr. Heinstein when he developed the leukemia because that really wasn't in my area of expertise. I'm more of an infectious disease physician. My area of expertise is AIDS/HIV. His subsequent problems have necessitated that we work with many different specialists because, as you know, at this point HIV is a disease that affects many different organs and one person can't really be responsible for all the parts of Frankie's care. I think that I have a slightly different perspective than Dr. Heinstein does in the sense that although many of the parts of Frankie's current disease are treatable in isolation, I have to wonder if he does have a cardiac arrest that requires resuscitation, given all the many different problems he has, what the final outcome would be if we resuscitate him.

*Bioethics mediator:* Could we hold the resuscitation discussion just for now. Again, what I hear you saying—and this is a hard one, so please make sure I have it right—is that he is very sick. He's got HIV disease, which has had a complicated course, and he now has leukemia, which has a complicated course. Can you give us some sense of how these two layer on each other? What does it mean to Frankie as a person, from your perspective as an HIV specialist, to have these two things together?

*The mediator does three things: She summarizes what Dr. Schwartz has said about the medical facts. She again puts off discussion about resuscitating Frankie. Then she asks a clarifying question that directs the focus back to the patient. By asking, "What does it mean to Frankie as a person?" she reminds all of the participants that this is not just a theoretical discussion; it concerns a real person.*

*Dr. Schwartz:* I would just like to add also the renal disease, which is significant in terms of his prognosis.

*Bioethics mediator:* And is that a result of his HIV?

*Dr. Schwartz:* They are all connected. The cardiac disease, the kidney disease, they really are all part of the same problem. It's very difficult to separate the causes and really not as important as understanding that there are many different things happening to him at the same time, each of which has a grave prognosis, which makes the hopefulness of his leaving the hospital very slim.

*Mr. Abruzzi:* So you think it probably doesn't make sense to resuscitate him?

*Bioethics mediator:* Well, again, Mr. Abruzzi, if you would just bear with me for a minute, we will get to the decision about resuscitation. I just want you to have a feeling of what the physicians are saying. I think what Dr. Schwartz is saying is that he has HIV disease, which he has had for a long time. That's related to his cardiac disease, which is now a free-standing problem. It's also related to his kidney disease. He's had one kidney removed and the other isn't working, and he now has leukemia. So what I hear from Dr. Schwartz actually is a bit of a different presentation than from Dr. Heinstein. That is, he has all of these things happening at once, which is a little bit different from Dr. Heinstein, who is focusing on his leukemia. We will get to the DNR discussion, if you would just bear with me.

*The mediator responds to Mr. Abruzzi's question by slowing things down. She again summarizes what the doctors have been saying. Then she explains why she is proceeding as she has been before asking him to wait on the DNR discussion. It would have been helpful also to acknowledge how difficult it is for parents to be faced with this decision.*

*Note the way the mediator presented the differences between the two doctors. She did not mention the word "disagreement"; instead she said they had made different presentations.*

*Mr. Abruzzi:* Whom do you agree more with?

*Bioethics mediator:* I don't agree or disagree with either of the physicians. I would only point out that they seem to be focusing on different aspects of Frankie's illness. That is not surprising. Dr. Heinstein is an oncologist, a specialist in the treatment of cancer. He is addressing this aspect of Frankie's illness which he was asked to do. Dr. Heinstein is really focused now on the leukemia, as he should be. He's an oncologist and we brought him in as a specialist to look at this problem. Let us see first what the different perspectives of the physicians are and then see whether or not they disagree.

*The mediator provides a bit of stroking for Dr. Heinstein by saying he is doing his job as a specialist. She preserves her neutrality by saying she does not agree or disagree with the doctors and brings some clarity to their differences by beginning to point out their different perspectives. Again, it would have been helpful to acknowledge Mr. Abruzzi's feelings.*

*Mr. Abruzzi:* That's not exactly what I'm talking about. I don't disagree that the deck is stacked against my son, but as long as there is one live card left to play, I think it's wrong for us not to play it. But even if you try dialysis, we still think resuscitation is wrong.

*Bioethics mediator:* That was very helpful. The only thing I would ask you is to leave words like right and wrong out because that won't help us. Your perspective, I think, is very clear, and, I think, very helpful. So can we put the DNR discussion aside for just a minute? So, two slightly different perspectives: one from our specialist whom we brought in—"Let's get this leukemia under control. I think we can." And Dr. Schwartz, who seems to be saying there are so many problems going on that it might not help to look only at the leukemia. Is that a fair statement Dr. Schwartz?

*The mediator again diverts the discussion from talk about the solution and returns to clarifying the issues.*

*The mediator's request that Mr. Abruzzi "leave words like right and wrong out because that won't help us" could be problematic on several counts. The statement could feel like a criticism to the parents, although framing it as a request mitigates the risk. Probably a more important problem with the statement is that the reason for it is unclear. The mediator was trying to remove from the table the notion that choices can be "right" or "wrong" but would have done so more effectively by saying something such as, "The goal of the mediation is to make decisions that feel 'right' to all."*

*Also, rather than sticking to her agenda, the mediator might have allowed the discussion temporarily to move in a different direction by exploring the "it would be wrong" statement by the father. She might have asked a clarifying question such as, "When you say it would be wrong, what do you mean?" and then again reassure the parents with a statement such as, "The goal of the mediation is to make decisions that feel 'right' to all."*

*Dr. Schwartz:* That and I guess my question about even if we can control many of these problems medically, what it's going to mean to Frankie who is the person that we're trying to treat.

*Bioethics mediator:* Maybe it would be helpful to get two other perspectives before we go on to talk about where we go with this. [Turning to Nurse Aquino:] You are the nurse caring for the patient?

*The mediator missed an opportunity to respond to Dr. Schwartz's comment following her earlier reminder that the focus needs to be on Frankie. She could have responded, "Maybe it would be helpful to get two other perspectives on what all of this means for Frankie."*

*Nurse Aquino:* Yes. I'm in the ICU. There are a group of us who care for the patients there, but I care for Frankie.

*Bioethics mediator:* And you've known him now since he's been in the ICU?

*Nurse Aquino:* Yes.

*Bioethics mediator:* Would you like to add anything?

*After a few narrow questions to the nurse, the mediator asks an open question.*

*Nurse Aquino:* I think that what we've been really struck with is the anguish that Mr. and Mrs. Abruzzi have been going through trying to make a decision. We see them there at the bedside, and we know that they're hearing different things from different people, and we know that they really love Frankie and they are really trying to make the very best decision for him. The nurses just feel that there is not enough for them to grapple with to make the decision that they're going to have to live with, no matter what happens to Frankie, whether he has a DNR or doesn't, whether he has treatment or not. They need to feel comfortable in their decision. I think the other thing is that the nurses are struggling with it too because we're there every day with Frankie. Mr. and Mrs. Abruzzi are there a lot of the time, but we're there 24 hours a day. We're taking care of Frankie and bathing him and taking care of all of his needs. We know that some of these decisions are going to have real consequences for us as the primary care givers. So we're really concerned about making sure that this is a decision that everybody understands.

*This is a terrific response from the nurse that everyone—including doctors and mediator—could learn from. Aquino begins by acknowledging the parents' feelings and recognizing their love for their son. She frames the issue as needing to give them enough information so that they can both make the decision (this is a statement of the issue) and live with it, whatever it is (this is a statement of their underlying interest). She then indicates her interests and those of the other nurses as the 24-hour-a-day caregivers.*

*Bioethics mediator:* You're lucky you have such good nurses. That makes a real difference. But I think that, Ms. Aquino, you raised a very important point, which is what I hope comes out of these discussions is not that they will have to make a decision but that we'll all reach an agreement that we're comfortable with so that we won't put all of that responsibility on them. [Turning to the parents:] Obviously, you have the authority to make decisions for Frankie—you're his parents. I think it's a very important point that, at best, we try to share the burdens of those decisions. Mr. Chen, do you have anything to add?

*The mediator acknowledges the value of the nurse's contribution and builds on her framing of the issue. She reassures Frankie's parents that the goal is to have the treatment team provide support for their decision making while recognizing the parents' ultimate authority. Then she invites the ICU social worker to join the discussion.*

*Mr. Chen:* Yes. We've talked in the ICU. I'm the social worker for the ICU. I see many situations like this, and I talked to the Abruzzis. We talked at length about

Frankie. From their point of view, they have a lot of feelings, obviously, about what's gone on to date. The sense that I got from talking to them is how overwhelming the situation is with their son and how unexpected all of these things are. He went into the ICU and now one of the things that hasn't been mentioned, but I think should be, is that he is now on a breathing machine too and he's not even conscious. He got dialysis and Mr. and Mrs. Abruzzi came into the ICU and they were really shocked to see all of this. I can understand that. So we talked a lot about their feelings and their dismay and their anguish and their sense of hopelessness because of all these things that are going on. It didn't seem like it would be this bad initially. They shared with me that they really wonder if Frankie is ever going to get better, and that maybe it's time to say, "Look, there's nothing more that we can do," and just let Frankie go in peace. I heard their saying that, and I can sympathize with that feeling. I can really see how under the circumstances they could really feel that way. So I've met with them frequently. They are going through a very difficult time and are confused about what to do. I think that's very understandable.

*The social worker adds more to the picture of what Mr. and Mrs. Abruzzi are going through. In a sense he speaks for them, saying things about what they are feeling that they might find difficult to say in a group. While mediators encourage parties to speak for themselves, there are times when they are unable or reluctant to do so and when having an advocate or surrogate speak for them is essential to having the process work.*

*Note that important information does not always come from the expected source. Here the social worker brought out an important medical fact—that the patient was on a ventilator—a fact that was not mentioned by either of the doctors or the nurse.*

*Bioethics mediator:* I wanted to make one more comment. [Turning to the risk manager:] Ms. Henry, I'm not exactly sure why you're here, but let me just make one comment based on what Mr. Chen said. In my role in this hospital over the last 25 years I've observed that hospitals are very good at making decisions to go ahead with treatment. They are not as good at making decisions to stop. One of the things that happened in bioethics discussions over the past years—the past decade really—is the sense that the perspective that maybe it's time to stop has to be of equal importance in these discussions. We're here to care for the whole patient and if the patient isn't going to make it, it's our obligation to recognize that and support a process of dying. So we're trying to figure out in the first instance whether we are at that point. So, let me just ask Ms. Henry why she's here and then let's sum up where we are. Then I think it's time to ask Dr. Schwartz to give us a summary of where you think we are and then begin to open the discussion of what our options are and how you might arrange those options. Does that make sense?

*The mediator is doing several things here. She realizes she needs to acknowledge the presence of the risk manager and allow her to speak. But before doing so, she draws on her expertise and experience, noting that it is harder to stop treatment than to go on treating and stating an ethical norm, that the obligation is to care for the whole patient and support the process of dying if that is what is called for. This is a rich and sophisticated move by the mediator. With this statement she does three things at once: she reminds all participants of the ethical norm; in a non-confrontational manner, she provides reality testing for the risk manager; and she reminds the risk manager that the mediator has been around long enough to know the games that get played in the hospital. The mediator's statement provides a helpful frame for the risk manager's comments and also a powerful hint about what kind of comments will be helpful.*

*The way the mediator's question to the risk manager is phrased, however, highlights a potentially inappropriate exchange. In many situations, a mediator may disagree with the stance of one of the parties. Risk managers are concerned above all with the hospital's liability, not necessarily with what is best for a particular patient. Nonetheless, it would have been inappropriate for this mediator to address the risk manager in an openly hostile way.*

*The mediator's comments suggest she feels that what she has heard so far points to a DNR order. From information she gathered before the mediation, she had a working hypothesis that continued treatment would be an extraordinary burden on Frankie and that the parents wanted a DNR but had been talked out of it by the oncologist. Rather than stating her view of the situation and then trying to sell the solution, she works with all the participants to help them reach a solution on their own.*

*At the end of this intervention the mediator gives a road map for the next part of the discussion: hear from the risk manager; get a summary of the current status from Dr. Schwartz; then discuss options and how those options might work. The road map gives all the participants time to think about what will happen next. Also, by asking Dr. Schwartz to speak about the current situation, she is giving him rather than Dr. Heinstein control of the next part of the discussion. This is a vivid example of the type of choices mediators make throughout a mediation. Any time a mediator steps in to summarize or clarify, he or she makes choices about to whom to direct the next question.*

*The mediator does not limit choices by saying the group will discuss the DNR order but, instead, invites a broader discussion of possible solutions, saying they will discuss options. In addition she coaches the participants on how to make the discussion of options productive when she suggests talking about what has to happen to make the options occur ("how to arrange the options").*

*This transcript does not pick up the way the mediator speaks or uses body language. By tone of voice she cultivates an air of uncertainty—not about what she is doing but about the situation being discussed. For example, her voice goes up at the end of sentences so that she does not seem to be lecturing. She creates a feeling of "Listen. I'm struggling with this just as much as you are." While she is clearly in control of this mediation, she does not impose her choices on the participants. She uses phrases such as "Does that make sense?" or "Is that OK?" She also uses eye contact to check with the family during the fact-gathering phase. The techniques she uses are designed to bring all of the participants along with her on the journey toward collaborative decision making.*

*Mediators and conflict resolvers need to be most tentative when they are making their most powerful moves. Being tentative keeps the mediator from coming across as the heavy; it gives participants choices; and it lets them know that they do not have to follow the mediator's lead.*

*The mediator in this case has kept the discussion focused on the medical situation, not on what should happen for Frankie. By spending so much time clarifying the medical facts she is empowering the parents, the ultimate decision makers, by providing them with information, by assuring them that they will have control over the ultimate decision, and by assuring them that the medical team—or at least most of the team members—will support them as they make a wrenching decision. Also, by using lay language in many of her summaries she enhances the likelihood that the parents will understand what the treatment team is saying. Similarly, by stating the ethical norms, the mediator is leveling the playing field between the family members who are wrestling with these issues for the first time and the members of the treatment team who have dealt with such situations before. Certainly there are limits to the effort to level the field, since the family does not have the experience to interpret the medical facts. But providing them with information about medical facts and governing standards can help the family members feel well enough informed to be more comfortable making the hard decision.*

**Bioethics mediator:** Dr. Schwartz, I'm going to come back to you in a minute to give us a summary, and if you can bear with us one more moment Mr. and Mrs. Abruzzi, I know that Ms. Henry is here and she sometimes has some very useful perspectives to add.

**Ms. Henry** (to the parents): We haven't met before, and the mediator asked initially why I was here. The risk manager's job is to make sure that decisions that are made are in keeping with hospital policy and with state law. Most of the time there is no problem, but sometimes in difficult situations there can be. In a situation like this where we're talking about possibly limiting the right to treatment, it's helpful sometimes for me to know what's going on and for me to be able to help you to know what the requirements are.

*Bioethics mediator:* Ms. Henry, just a point. Thank you for being here. You and I have worked together for a long time and I think it's helpful to have the administration which Ms. Henry represents as part of the discussion. And, Ms. Henry, you know that I respect those issues a lot, but again, can we put them aside for a minute? But let me make my perspective on this case clear. Mr. and Mrs. Abruzzi are the family of the patient and we're going to look in a bit at what the patient would want and what they would want, but it's very clear to me that they have the legal right to make this decision and the moral right to make it. I understand, and thank you for being here because it will be helpful for you to hear their perspective, but I don't think there's any question in this case. As Frankie's parents, they really do have the right to make the decision.

*The mediator validates the risk manager's contribution but goes on to state, in very strong terms, a position about who has the legal and ethical right to make decisions in this case. In doing so she is fulfilling an institutional responsibility and is being highly evaluative on this point.*

*Given the behavior of the risk manager thus far in the mediation, the mediator's laying down the law about who will be the decision makers seems too strong. No doubt the mediator and the risk manager have a history, which moves the mediator to, in effect, make a pre-emptive strike. Doing so may keep the risk manager in line, but it may also make it hard for her to become part of the problem-solving team and it creates the risk that she will not buy into whatever agreement is reached. In addition, the highly evaluative intervention may send a message to the other participants that undermines their understanding of the mediator's role as someone who is there to facilitate a resolution. Such an evaluative intervention suggests that the mediator is perfectly prepared to be a judge and this suggestion may undermine the trust that she has been establishing with the other participants.*

*The mediator's strong assertion to the risk manager may reflect the fact that in New York State, the site of this mediation, case law would limit decisions to withdraw or withhold care from a decisionally incapacitated patient to those instances in which the previously capable patient had left explicit instructions, by clear and convincing evidence. But there is an exception if physicians say that the care is not medically appropriate. Here the parents' attempt to withhold dialysis could trigger this very restrictive surrogate analysis that the courts have suggested, or*

*the physician could say that the patient is no longer appropriate for this interven-*
*tion, which would shift the burden of the decision from the parents back to the*
*physician. This case provides a good example of the fact that usually a bioethics*
*mediator must know the relevant state law. In New York the discussion about*
*decision making for incapacitated patients must always be held in the context of*
*the case law. Bioethics professionals tend to be dismayed by the narrow empower-*
*ment of surrogates in the state and to work to reframe the situation to avoid trig-*
*gering these concerns; risk managers tend to give greater weight to these legal*
*analyses.*

   *In many hospitals it is common to have the risk manager participate in bioethics*
*mediations. The risk manager's presence here adds a potential legal dimension to*
*the discussion. The mediator must keep the discussion focused on the need for de-*
*cision making and not let it turn into a debate about legal principles.*

**Ms. Henry:** Well, we need to talk a little bit about limiting life-sustaining treatment
in the absence of knowing what the patient would want.

**Bioethics mediator:** If we need to. But we may not in this case. So let's go on to Dr.
Schwartz. Sum up for us how you would characterize medically what's happening now.

   *Rather than getting into a battle with the risk manager about the legal issues, the*
*mediator acknowledges her point but defers discussion of it and returns to Dr.*
*Schwartz for his summary. Here again the mediator's choice to defer an issue that*
*may derail discussion keeps the mediation on track.*

**Dr. Schwartz:** Well, I think Frankie has multiple organs involved in his disease. He's
currently on a respirator. He has many conditions in and of themselves that
could be treated and if he had them alone, there would be the possibility of successful treatment. Although none of us can really predict what the outcome of
serious illness is, in cases like Frankie's, I think it would be very unusual if he
were to be able to leave the hospital.

**Bioethics mediator:** So if I hear you correctly, you think that Frankie, given all of
the problems with the different parts of his body and different organ systems,
would it be too much to say that you think he may be in the process of dying?

   *The mediator summarizes in simpler language and uses the word "dying" rather*
*than the euphemisms used by the doctor. Doing so accomplishes two things. First,*
*her summary puts the reality of Frankie's situation clearly on the table. Second, it*
*lets the mediator test whether Dr. Schwartz can accept the characterization that*
*this patient is in the process of dying, a strong characterization that even some*
*doctors who would permit the DNR order would not be willing to accept. This*

*mediator used the most extreme characterization of Frankie's condition because she felt that whether Dr. Schwartz agreed with it would, to a large extent, determine the direction of the rest of the discussion.*

**Dr. Schwartz:** No. I think that's a fair statement.

**Bioethics mediator:** OK. I think we really need now to begin to grapple with what we're going to do. We've heard two very different things. We have two views here and in both cases, I think, Dr. Schwartz and Dr. Heinstein, you both agree the probabilities are not great, but we've heard Dr. Heinstein say, "We can treat the leukemia," and we've heard Dr. Schwartz say, "Even if we treat the leukemia, it may be that he's just overwhelmed by all of the medical things that are happening." So you, Dr. Schwartz, think it's OK to stop and you [Dr. Heinstein] think you shouldn't. It's OK to keep on going. Mr. and Mrs. Abruzzi, which of those interpretations seems to make more sense to you? How have you experienced his care here and how are you thinking about what's happening?

*As the mediator turns the discussion to problem solving, she is clear and direct: the doctors agree that Frankie's chances are not very good. Their views differ about what should be the next steps in Frankie's treatment.*

*After her summary, the mediator turns to the parents. She asks multiple questions ("Which of those interpretations seems to make more sense to you? How have you experienced his care here and how are you thinking about what's happening?"). In general, asking multiple questions can be problematic, but here, where the parents have been waiting for the opportunity to speak and may be uncertain about what they want to say, using multiple questions invites them to choose from a range of topics, starting where they are most comfortable, while still providing some guidance about the structure of the discussion.*

*These parents are being asked to make difficult decisions. They know that the doctors disagree and therefore they might fear that they are being asked to choose between the two doctors, both of whose care is important for their son. While the mediator does not hide the differences, she first emphasizes the common ground— that they agree on the overall medical picture. (She actually catches herself starting with their differences: "We've heard two different things. We have two views here . . ." Then she realizes that it would be better to point out the common ground and says, ". . . and in both cases, I think Dr. Schwartz and Dr. Heinstein, you both agree the probabilities are not great," before being specific about their differing views concerning treatment.)*

*This way of summarizing helps the parents see that even though the doctors have strong feelings about their differences, they are both committed to Frankie and, in fact, are really not very far apart. A clearer summary that stressed the doc-*

tors' agreement about the general prognosis and made clear that in addition to being committed to Frankie, each doctor wants what he thinks is best for Frankie might have made the parents' decision-making task easier.

*Mrs. Abruzzi:* Well, I just see him being more and more overwhelmed. Every time I come in there are more tubes in him. He's not at all responsive. I just don't want him in pain anymore.

*Bioethics mediator:* Well, let me assure you, just on that issue, that we take the treatment of pain as an ethical issue, not just as a medical issue. There are studies now that show that 55 percent of the patients who die, die in pain. On our team we think that is ethically unacceptable. And so, I think we can get agreement from Dr. Schwartz and the ICU nurses that he will not be in any pain, that he will have a level of sedation and analgesia that will keep him comfortable. Do you have any problems with that?

*The mediator responds to the mother's concern about pain with direct information, which both reassures the parents and takes that issue off the table. After she makes her statement about pain treatment, the mediator checks with the parents to see whether they have any additional concern about pain management.*

*Mr. Abruzzi:* No.

*Bioethics mediator:* All right. So let's put that one aside. We promise you that he will not suffer and be in pain. That's a medical issue, and a nursing issue.

*Mrs. Abruzzi:* It's just hard because he's gone through so much. He's a real fighter. There's absolutely no question about it. It's hard because now when we come in we see him unconscious with all these tubes. It's just very distressing.

*Bioethics mediator:* Tell us a little bit about Frankie. You say he's a fighter. It's real important for this discussion not just because he's your son and you love him but I'm going to suggest to you that as we move on to figure out together what to do, what he would want is very important. So who he is and what he wants is really a critical next piece of the discussion, so tell us something about him.

*The mediator does some active listening, reflecting not only what Mrs. Abruzzi has said about Frankie being a fighter but also her feelings, her love for her son. She is inviting the parents to introduce the whole Frankie, not just Frankie the patient, to the mediator and to the other participants. She also explains that knowing what Frankie would want is important to the decision making and to them.*

*Regardless of whether the mediation involves just the medical team or the team and the family, it is important that the mediator provide an opportunity for the patient to be introduced to her. The "introduction" can be done by the family or the family and members of the treatment team. Making sure the absent patient is introduced has several values: it reminds everyone of why they are there; it assures family members of the medical team's concern; it may provide important information about what this patient would want; it may help the family members clarify their thinking and help them separate their own emotional reactions from decisions about what the patient would want; and it humanizes the decision-making process.*

*When the mediator turned to the parents she made a critical change in the direction of the discussion. She shifted from objectively gathering medical information to considering the parents' concerns and how Frankie might approach the difficult decision.*

*Mr. Abruzzi:* Well, he had a rough life. He has HIV and a problem with his heart and then the cancer. For a lot of people that would just mean depression, that would just mean a sense that your life is over. He's never been like that. These have been really tough obstacles for him, but he's gone on and tried to live and enjoy life. He's the type of person that sees the bright side in everything. He's a real joy and he's a very hopeful person. Obstacles have never slowed him down. It's been very hard to see him unconscious here because we don't see that side of him. It's almost like when he's unconscious he's not here anymore. Part of me says, if he were just awake now he'd be saying, "I'll get through this, Dad. Don't worry about it." He's just strong that way. Seeing him now is just like he's not there. He's a real fighter.

*Mrs. Abruzzi:* I'm sorry. Could I share my perspective of Frankie as a person?

*Bioethics mediator:* Sure. I just wanted to understand something from Mr. Abruzzi and then that would be very helpful. Mr. Abruzzi, it sounds to me like you're saying that if you ran a summer camp you would want Frankie in your bunk. He's a really good, optimistic guy. As his illness went on, did he keep that optimism? So he wanted to have his kidney removed because he thought that was the next step, and he agreed to start dialysis. Let me rephrase the question. When his other kidney began to malfunction and he knew this was a whole new ball game, he was still making decisions about his care, and he wanted to go ahead and get the machine that would supplant his kidney, the dialysis machine. He wanted to do that?

*The bioethics mediator continues talking to Mr. Abruzzi even though Mrs. Abruzzi has asked for an opportunity to speak about Frankie. While what the mediator wanted to ask was valuable, she could have waited and allowed Mrs. Abruzzi into the discussion.*

*The language used by the mediator as she summarizes what she has heard from the parents about Frankie ("If you ran a summer camp. . . . He's a really good, op-*

*timistic guy.") shows the parents that she has developed an appreciation for Frankie the person and sees him as more than a patient.*

**Mr. Abruzzi:** Yes.

**Bioethics mediator:** For me, that's really important because one of the things when a patient can't make a decision, like Frankie clearly can't, we try to figure out with you what he would want. That's our first step. What would he want? Has he told us anything? Has he said anything specific, or has his behavior indicated anything? So that's really important. Dr. Heinstein, is there something you wanted to say about what Frankie would want?

*Here the mediator reiterates the guiding principle for the way decisions are made for unconscious patients: the patient's own wishes are important and must be taken seriously. The goal is to do what the patient would want to do, and if that cannot be determined, then the discussion becomes what is best for the patient. Setting out this guideline is an example of the bioethics mediator's norm-establishing role.*

*But note that the mother has still not had the opportunity, which she requested, to speak about Frankie.*

**Dr. Heinstein:** Just two things. It was months ago when I made the diagnosis of leukemia. At that time, he did not have a do not resuscitate order. He did know he had the diagnosis of both HIV and the leukemia.

**Bioethics mediator:** He did know?

**Dr. Heinstein:** Of course he did. At the point at which he had the renal failure and had to have the nephrectomy, he wanted everything done. So the family and all of us thought that dialysis would be a good way to go because Frankie was such a fighter. I totally agree with that. My only problem right now is that of the options we have, the do not resuscitate, the dialysis, and the treatment for leukemia. We don't have a chance to treat any of those, and I think Frankie would want us to try something.

**Bioethics mediator:** That was very helpful. Let me tell you why I found that helpful, and tell me if you agree. Dr. Heinstein just identified three choices we have to make. One is whether to continue dialysis, two is whether to have a DNR order, and three is whether to treat the leukemia. OK. Let's say that those are the three choices we now have to make because that's helpful to me because it tells us where we have to go. I think that the piece about what Frankie would want is very helpful. So Dr. Heinstein is saying that as long as he could make decisions by himself he went ahead. Patients, if they are lucky, have a loving family to make decisions. So when you were all making that decision together, which I assume you did, he wanted to go ahead, whatever the chances. So he wanted to go ahead with the nephrectomy when he had his kidney removed, and he wanted to go ahead with the treatment of his leukemia. And you supported that with him.

*Parents:* Absolutely.

*Bioethics mediator:* So my question to you now would be, do you think he would change his mind now and why, or maybe, Mr. Abruzzi, if there is a chance, as Dr. Heinstein says, that maybe the leukemia will get better and maybe he'll get over this crisis—which Dr. Schwartz is not sure of. Part of the problem in medicine is we don't know what's going to happen. We can't give you promises that if you take route A this will be fine. We can't tell you that. So there's a lot of uncertainty, but I want to know whether you think Frankie would want to go ahead now with the leukemia treatment, because I think that is the key issue. If we go ahead with the leukemia treatment, then at least for the moment, it doesn't make sense to have the DNR. [To Dr. Heinstein:] In other words, if we're going to go ahead with the leukemia treatment, the DNR doesn't make sense. Is that your position?

*The mediator asks the parents to consider whether, given what has happened, Frankie would change his mind about wanting further leukemia treatment and acknowledges how difficult it is to make decisions under conditions of uncertainty. She then gives them a moment to sit with the question before asking for a response. In the meantime she clarifies the choice that needs to be made with a question to Dr. Heinstein.*

*Dr. Heinstein:* More accurately, I think we should at least do the treatment whether we have the DNR or not. We should at least do the treatment.

*Bioethics mediator:* So you think you can separate those two?

*Dr. Heinstein:* I can separate them, although my preference for Frankie and what I think is the better position is no do not resuscitate order, given the fact that everything that's happened to him is reversible.

*The mediator's clarifying question narrows the decision that needs to be made. The choice is no longer between treating the leukemia and signing a DNR order. Dr. Heinstein acknowledges that it is possible to do both, though he still opposes the DNR.*

*Bioethics mediator:* So you would agree, too, that there are three decisions, and they are separate. One is whether to go ahead with his dialysis, which isn't an issue now because, as I understand it, he's too sick. But, if we went ahead with the leukemia treatment—that's decision one—it might put him in a position where we could institute dialysis. That would be decision two, and then the DNR is a separate decision. Dr. Schwartz, does it make sense to you to look at those three decisions separately?

*Dr. Schwartz:* Well, yes. I'm not uncomfortable doing that. I think that they can be separated.

*Once again the mediator slows the process down, breaks the decisions into parts, and gets both doctors to agree on the way she characterizes what needs to be decided. Having done this, she turns to the mother, who had earlier asked for an opportunity to be heard.*

*Bioethics mediator:* OK. Good. So now let's come back to Frankie. What do you think he wants? What would he want?

*Mrs. Abruzzi:* I'm not sure what he would want, but he's a fighter. His father's right about that. I wouldn't want him to be in any pain.

*Bioethics mediator:* But remember, we will not let him be in any pain.

*Mrs. Abruzzi:* You're sure about that?

*Bioethics mediator:* Absolutely. Absolutely. Has he ever talked about other people who were in a similar situation, either people he knew, people in the family who were critically ill. Has he ever talked about their treatment?

*Mrs. Abruzzi:* No.

*Bioethics mediator:* So let's again put that aside for now.

*Mrs. Abruzzi:* So there's no pain, even when he's unconscious with the tubes and everything. It's so hard. When somebody can talk they can tell you. You can see it on their face. You can see it in their reaction. When they just have tubes in them and they are unconscious it's hard.

*What is happening here happens often in mediations. Although the discussion has moved ahead, options have been generated, and the time has come to begin making decisions, Mrs. Abruzzi has concerns about Frankie's pain, which she has raised twice before, that need to be explored and addressed before she can participate in the decision making.*

*Bioethics mediator:* Nurse Aquino, could you talk a little bit to us about how nurses figure out when a patient is in pain? I agree with you. That for me is the most important ethical issue. So I think it would be helpful if the family understood how the nursing team reacts to pain.

*Despite assurances from the mediator, Mrs. Abruzzi continues to be anxious about pain management. Even though for purposes of what needs to happen during the mediation, this is not an issue, the mother's concern is getting in the way of the mediator's efforts to focus on the three decisions she has identified. The mediator recognizes the need to deal with Mrs. Abruzzi's concerns before trying to move on and asks for information from an expert, the ICU nurse.*

*In a situation like this, when a party keeps raising a concern that the mediator thinks has been addressed, it is often a good idea to invite the party to talk more about it. Here the mediator might have acknowledged the mother's concern by saying something like, "Mrs. Abruzzi, you've mentioned your worry that Frankie is in pain. I have the sense that even though we've promised that the nurses are sensitive to this issue and will do what is needed to keep Frankie pain free, you still have concerns about it. Maybe we haven't been clear about what is being done for Frankie. In a minute I'm going to ask Ms. Aquino to explain more about how his pain is being managed, but first, could you tell us a little more about what is worrying you?" Giving Mrs. Abruzzi the opportunity to talk about her concern about Frankie's pain might have helped her clarify her own fears and would also have told Nurse Aquino what information would be most helpful to Mrs. Abruzzi.*

*Nurse Aquino:* Well, I think we try to do a couple of things. First, I think just what you're saying. When people have tubes, the assumption would be that they are experiencing pain, just like anybody else. So we start from that perspective. We want to make sure that the pain is treated. We treat the pain, but also every time we turn Frankie, every time we try, we have to sometimes take out the fluid through his nose and suction him, we look to see if he flinches. We look to see if he grimaces in any way. We look to see if we have any evidence at all that he's in pain. And, we've gotten pretty good at knowing that. You're right. It's not like having the person tell us directly. Obviously, it's not the same, but we're experienced. We're here all the time, and we're pretty good at trying to judge. Working with Dr. Schwartz and the other doctors, this is an ICU where if we're in doubt, we treat the pain. We don't say, "Well these people aren't experiencing pain because they are unconscious." We are really up on all the latest stuff and we really try to treat the pain. The doctors and nurses are in agreement about that.

*Dr. Schwartz:* I just wanted to add that what you are feeling is pain, and it's a different kind of pain than you are worried about Frankie feeling. So when you see him with all these tubes, you have to separate your pain as parents from his physical pain as a patient.

*Nurse Aquino:* But that's what I was going to say. Sometimes parents identify so much with their children that their own suffering, they think that because they are suffering their children are suffering too. And that's not the case here.

*Bioethics mediator:* I think you can be comfortable that, despite the terrible level of anguish and pain that you two have, he will not experience physical pain. So, are you comfortable on that point?

*Both nurse and doctor validate the parent's feeling by recognizing their emotional pain while giving additional information about the treatment of Frankie's pain. The mediator summarizes that Frankie is not in physical pain, adds her acknowledgment of the parents' suffering, and checks to see whether they are ready to move on.*

*Mrs. Abruzzi:* Yes.

*Mr. Abruzzi:* That was very helpful.

*Bioethics mediator:* OK. That's a very important point. So now let's come back because I think there is a very important issue here. Let me state to you what I know here. Frankie's a fighter. Every time he reached a juncture where he could make a decision to go ahead and be treated, he did. That's a really important thing. If we want to try to make the decision for him now that he would make, that's very powerful evidence. Dr. Heinstein is saying that's his sense of Frankie also. So, let me try to break up these three decisions in the order in which they seem to make sense. One is to go ahead in treating the leukemia. But let me tell you what I hear. I hear from the two of you that if Frankie could make the decision, he might make the decision to go ahead. But that's pretty important. I would argue to you now that if that's the decision that he would make, maybe that's the decision we should make.

*The mediator demonstrates a key mediator skill—patience. She takes time to reiterate what she has heard about Frankie's being a fighter; she states the governing principle for making this decision—that it be what he would choose for himself if he were able—and only then does she present the hypothesis ("I would argue . . .") that if Frankie were in a condition to do so, he would chose treatment for the leukemia. Here again the written transcript does not reflect the way the mediator's tone of voice softens the word "argue" and makes it clear she is only putting out a hypothesis.*

*Mrs. Abruzzi:* Oh sure. We're OK with that.

*Bioethics mediator:* OK. So we're moving along. Dr. Heinstein. Dr. Schwartz, are you comfortable with that?

*The parents agree with the hypothesis. The mediator characterizes what is happening as progress, then checks with the two doctors.*

*Dr. Schwartz:* I am. I think that I am here to try to represent Frankie's needs. I think we all are, and it's important that we get at them.

*Bioethics mediator:* OK. So I think we're moving. As I said to you, my goal doesn't always work. I've had some spectacular failures, but my role is always to try to get everyone to be comfortable with the decision because then nobody feels the burden exclusively. So let's say that we're going to go ahead with treating the leukemia. Dr. Heinstein, let me argue with you a little bit. The parents would like the leukemia treated, and my guess is that if you asked them, they would probably do it. But it's pretty problematic. Even you would agree that this is a very sick patient. Treating the leukemia may not work. The patient is already intubated, so if there is a pulmonary event, if something happens in his lungs, he is not really going to go into arrest. So the question is, if under the assault of everything that's happening in his body, if his heart stops, what should we do? I think that you might agree that if that happens and there is yet one more layer, that maybe it's appropriate to recognize that we and Frankie have lost this battle. I really ask you to reconsider. The parents are saying they would like you to treat the leukemia. Let's give it one more chance, but if he should arrest, let's be ready to accept that judgment. Could you live with that?

*The mediator tries some reality testing (she calls it arguing) with Dr. Heinstein. As she does so she draws on her own medical knowledge to try to focus on the realities of the case.*

*At one point the mediator starts to use a medical term, "pulmonary," but catches herself and switches to lay language, "if something happens in his lungs," which makes it easier for the parents to follow the discussion.*

*Dr. Heinstein:* I would accept it [the DNR] then, but I'm not entirely comfortable with that, again given my tradition that we should at least try to restart his heart.

*Bioethics mediator:* But your tradition is if there is any chance at all, you take it. Maybe the parents and Frankie come from a different tradition which is less powerful, and in a situation of so much uncertainty and anguish, it would not be unreasonable for them to make the decision that a cardiac arrest really was the end of this. The end of the life of their child.

*The mediator presses Dr. Heinstein. Two things seem to be going on in these exchanges. First, she is making arguments to test his position. Second, she is setting things up to give the parents permission to choose to stop treatment if that is what they want.*

*Mr. Abruzzi:* If my wife and I could just talk to each other for a moment. I appreciate you all being here because this has been very helpful. I was just wondering if we could just talk for a moment.

*Bioethics mediator:* Absolutely. Would you like some coffee. There is a coffee machine at the nurses' station. It makes the worst coffee in history, but I'm sure they'd be willing to share it with you. Do you want to go and get a cup of coffee and talk, and then you can come back and we'll talk some more.

[The parents leave the room. Once they do, the battle becomes much more confrontational.]

*During the debriefing of this mediation, the mediator noted that when members of a treatment team disagree about the appropriate course of treatment, she tries to have a preliminary meeting without the patient or family. In a staff-only meeting the conversation can be more direct. In this case Dr. Schwartz might have said, to Dr. Heinstein, "Come on. You've got to be kidding me. This guy is dying. One more day and putting him back on dialysis is really not going to help. Your talking to the family about the fact that this can happen is only confusing them and you know and I know that this patient is dying. Let's deal with this patient as a dying patient." It can be useful for the medical staff to have this kind of direct airing of the conflict, something that would not be helpful for the family. Once the parents left the room the mediator continued with a more direct approach.*

*Bioethics mediator:* Hey, what's bugging you about this case? I think we're moving nicely. The family is going to agree with treating the leukemia. Dr. Heinstein is going to agree.

*Dr. Schwartz:* We don't know why they wanted it.

*Bioethics mediator:* They want it because their son is dying.

*Dr. Schwartz:* You haven't heard from them why they want it.

*Bioethics mediator:* You said you could live with treating the cancer.

*Dr. Schwartz:* Well, I heard you say that you would only accept the DNR order if you couldn't do anything at all to help the patient.

*Dr. Heinstein:* So it sounds like you're backing away from that.

*Dr. Schwartz:* What are you trying to save? You know, if you resuscitate this guy, the chances of him regaining consciousness are .01 percent. He has a million other problems that are going on. This guy is not getting out of the hospital if he has another arrest. You're treating his bone marrow. You're not treating him.

*Bioethics mediator:* I think, Dr. Heinstein, that in the business of compromising on medical decisions and where we're going and what's happening, you've won this one. Give them a break. You've won it. You're going to go ahead. They're very uncertain, but they're with you. Give them a break on the DNR. We haven't come to that yet.

[The parents return.]

*Mrs. Abruzzi:* We were just listening to you before we went out to talk. The pain has really been my only concern. That's why I signed the DNR order. I didn't want him to be in pain. My husband has always not wanted to do that, but I have one more question about the DNR. If you do something and you resuscitate him, will he be in more pain? Will he hurt? Are you going to do things to him that will make things worse off?

*Bioethics mediator:* If his heart stops and we resuscitate him, or if we try—It's not clear that that will work, but if we try, would that add to his pain? Let's assume that he stays at the baseline that he is now. Could that cause additional pain?

*Dr. Schwartz:* It's possible, but again, not unmanageably. It could prolong it though. More than additional pain, it could take us longer and longer in an area of greater uncertainty.

*Mrs. Abruzzi:* But the act of resuscitating him wouldn't make him hurt a lot more?

*Dr. Heinstein:* He is unconscious already. If his heart stops and the blood ceases to flow to his brain, he is not going to feel any more pain. Yes, the resuscitation might not work.

*Mrs. Abruzzi:* The only thing we are worried about is his pain. If you're telling me that he's not going to be in more pain, then we're prepared to tear the DNR up for now.

*Bioethics mediator:* Dr. Heinstein, Dr. Schwartz, are we agreed that even if we try to resuscitate the patient, given his present medical condition, giving the alertness of the medical and nursing staff, that he will not experience more pain?

*Dr. Schwartz:* I don't think we can say it for sure. I think the thing is, after he's resuscitated, if he lives, we may be back to where we were, but we may be into a situation we've got other medical options that we have to try.

*Bioethics mediator:* But why would that increase his pain?

*Dr. Schwartz:* Because every time you have a new thing going on, it makes it harder to control the pain. That doesn't mean we wouldn't make every effort, and in most instances we're successful.

*Bioethics mediator:* This is hard for his parents to hear.

*Mr. Abruzzi:* But isn't he unconscious? Isn't that what Dr. Heinstein said?

*Dr. Schwartz:* But there are levels of pain that can be experienced even when the patient is unconscious.

*Bioethics mediator:* So deep pain. Can you leave an order for morphine that would be sufficient to control that eventuality?

*Dr. Schwartz:* Yes.

*Bioethics mediator:* OK. If your single concern is the pain issue, then Dr. Schwartz says he can leave an order that is sufficiently strong for pain medication. We can't promise you 100 percent in a package wrapped in gold. Medicine isn't that way. But we can promise you our best efforts. What I hear from you is that if we can do that then you would like to go ahead with the leukemia treatment for now. Remember, the decision we reached today we can all get back together and change tomorrow. But for today, where we are now, you would like Dr. Heinstein to continue with treating the leukemia, and you would like for the moment to suspend the DNR. Is that comfortable for you now?

*Mrs. Abruzzi:* Yes.

*Mr. Abruzzi:* Yes.

*Bioethics mediator:* Are we all in agreement? OK. I think we can end for now, although you have to understand, as we all do, that things change all the time, and we're available for you if you'd like to come back into the conversation. My guess is that everyone is on board; that we're going to try this. If this doesn't "work," if the leukemia doesn't get better, then I think Dr. Heinstein and you will be more comfortable knowing everything was tried, and then it will be a different discussion. But for now, are we all in agreement? OK. Thank you. Thank you very much for coming. I know this was a very hard decision, but I think you were very courageous to face it, and we think you're good advocates for your son.

*Mrs. Abruzzi:* Thank you.

*In her last two comments the mediator summarizes what the participants have agreed on—controlling pain, treating the leukemia, and suspending the DNR—and reminds the parents and the treatment team that the decision can be revisited and revised depending on how Frankie responds. She also validates the contribution of the parents to the decision-making process.*

## Further Discussion

The mediator entered this case with the working hypothesis that a DNR order was appropriate—a view that she still had at the end of the mediation. Because she was able to put her preconceptions aside, make sure that all the relevant facts were on the table, and listen to the participants, she avoided imposing her views and allowed the mediation process to lead to an outcome that was very different from the one she anticipated.

Some observers of this mediation were troubled by the decision to continue treatment because they viewed this as a futility case. (In New York State the definition of futility is either the treatment will not work—for example, using an antibiotic to treat a virus—or the patient will go into cardiac arrest repeatedly in a short period.) The observers in the mediation for Frankie's case thought that a DNR based on futility should have been written and that it was unethical to take up an ICU bed and continue to expose nurses to the risks of treating an HIV patient. The mediator's view was that these parents knew their son was dying but were not quite ready to face that fact. They needed to feel they had done everything they could for their son. Since the proposed treatment was not going to harm Frankie, the mediator did not see continued treatment as unethical. She anticipated that the resuscitation was not going to work but saw this treatment as being for the benefit of the parents, not the patient. She stated that when she is sure the patient is beyond pain, she sometimes thinks it is helpful to treat the family because doing so lets them live more comfortably afterward with the consequences of the decision.

Had any of the participants raised the futility issue the mediator would have explored it. The fact that no one on the treatment team saw the case that way determined the direction of the discussion. When one of the doctors or the nurses in a mediation says, "This resuscitation effort will be futile," the mediator will argue that it is the team's ethical obligation to write a futility order of DNR to avoid exposing staff unnecessarily to HIV infection.

Other observers were concerned that the mediator did not ask the parents whether they understood what the process of resuscitation entails. When the parents returned to the room they had decided on resuscitation and no one explained how violent resuscitation can be, that it might result in broken ribs, information that might be important for the parents, especially given the mother's concern about pain. The mediator explained that once the parents made the decision, she did not go further with the discussion. She assumed that if this patient's heart stopped, the staff would respond with a resuscitation attempt, and that no one was going to pursue this attempt over a long time. Her assumption was that if Frankie's heart stopped, the staff would make an attempt and they would be able to see pretty quickly whether it was successful and if it was not they would stop.

## Postscript

In January 1999, two years after the actual mediation, the mediator spoke with the oncologist in the real case on which this role play was based to get an update. The patient recovered enough to go on dialysis until he was able to leave the hospital without needing it. When asked, the patient made it clear that he would want everything done again if necessary. He was never told that his parents had initially signed a DNR order. At the time of the conversation between the mediator and the oncologist, the patient was still being treated for AIDS and it was under good control. He was working and still receiving interferon for his chronic leukemia, which was also under good control. The patient's mother has since died of cancer.

# Afterword

A WELL-STRUCTURED mediation program can resolve a current dispute and also prevent future problems. During often emotional and contentious discussions, the bioethics mediator acts as both coach and model while responding to highly charged statements and strongly held views. The way he or she asks questions, summarizes to show all participants that they have been heard, and rephrases statements to make it easier for participants to listen demonstrates for members of the treatment team how they might have communicated more clearly (or listened more attentively). In addition, mediators may provide explicit coaching for the team members as they discuss the history of the case, help them plan how to communicate issues and information to the patient or family, and consider how to avoid similar problems in the future.

Another benefit of mediation is that the mediator and the team members may become aware of policies or practices that led to, or at least contributed to, the conflict and can bring those insights to the organization's leaders. Finally, by analyzing statistics about bioethics disputes, the hospital management may identify patterns that indicate the need for more staff training or identify a unit that is not functioning well.

Bioethics consultants who have mastered mediation skills will find those skills useful in undertaking less formal interventions and in addressing problems at an early stage—especially problems with communication—before a full-scale conflict develops. And as hospital staff, through participation in mediation, develop trust in the mediators and respect for their skills, they will develop the habit of consulting the mediators when they see conflicts begin to develop.

The cultural and ethnic makeup of our society is becoming more and more diverse at the same time that advances in medicine are increasing both the complexity and the uncertainty in treatment. Therefore, establishing a process for airing and understanding different points of view and resolving differences over bioethical disputes—and those issues where all sorts of conflicts are hung on a bioethics peg—

in medical decision making becomes more and more important. Mediation offers the necessary structural supports for such a process.

Mediators provide a setting in which cultural values can be voiced and honored, in which differing patterns in language and communication can be identified and bridged, and in which the voices of patients and families from traditionally disempowered groups can be amplified. Differences in age, gender, professional training, language, religion, level of education, and preference for either a contextual framework or a linear argument can all complicate communications among patients, families, and medical personnel and contribute to miscommunication and conflict. In bioethics mediation, these differences can be identified and worked through until comfortable agreement is reached about a plan of care.

One of the values of mediation in resolving bioethics disputes is that it runs counter to the tradition of conflict, confrontation, and malpractice suits that are such disastrous elements of today's health care system. Mediation can produce better quality and more enduring decisions. Furthermore, clarifying facts and options for care is a critical step in delivering high-quality patient care. Fear of possible future legal consequences, lack of clarity about legal and ethical analyses, and uncertainty about the decision-making process preclude the sort of clear thinking and consideration that excellent patient care requires. We will have to await the outcome of studies on the effectiveness of mediation as compared with imposed solutions to demonstrate that these mediated conflicts produce patient care plans that are comfortable for all. For now anecdotal reports must suffice, and those indicate that the process of mediating bioethics disputes leaves patients, families, and staff satisfied that what they are doing is the best for the patient given the medical constraints.

It is our hope that the model presented will lead to increased collaboration between the medical and mediation worlds while continuing to help patients, families, and their health care providers craft shared solutions to medically and emotionally complex and wrenching health care decisions.

# Suggested Reading on Mediation

WE HAVE NOT ATTEMPTED to review the literature on bioethics consultation in this volume. For a full bibliography on bioethics consultation see American Society of Bioethics and Humanities 1998. Since there is no comparable compilation for the mediation literature as it relates to bioethics we have focused on that literature.

## Books

Arrow K, RH Mnookin, L Ross, A Tversky, and R Wilson, eds. 1995. *Barriers to conflict resolution*. New York: W. W. Norton. Elegant, theoretical discussion of barriers to agreement.

Bush RAB and JP Folger. 1994. *The promise of mediation: Responding to conflict through empowerment and recognition*. San Francisco: Jossey-Bass. Important and controversial book that argues that empowerment and recognition, rather than agreement, should be the basic goals of mediation and presents the techniques that promote those goals.

Cialdini R. 1993. *Influence: The psychology of persuasion*. New York: William Morrow. An entertaining presentation of significant psychological material.

Costantino C and C Merchant. 1996. *Designing conflict management systems*. San Francisco: Jossey-Bass.

Deutsch M. 1973. *The resolution of conflict*. New Haven: Yale University Press. A seminal work.

Deutsch M and PT Coleman, eds. 2000. *The handbook of conflict resolution: Theory and practice*. San Francisco: Jossey-Bass. Indispensable, accessible guide for those seeking a deeper understanding of conflict resolution theory.

Dubler NN and LJ Marcus. 1994. *Mediating bioethical disputes*. New York: United Hospital Fund.

Fadiman A. 1998. *The spirit catches you and you fall down: A Hmong child, her American doctors, and the collision of two cultures*. Paperback. New York: Farrar, Straus and Giroux. A story of cultural misunderstandings in a health care setting. Not directly related to mediation but a book everyone working with people from different cultures could learn from.

Fisher R and W Ury. 1981. *Getting to yes: Negotiating agreement without giving in*. Paperback. New York: Penguin. A classic. Presents the techniques for collaborative or "win-win" negotiation. In the mediation process, mediators assist parties to negotiate this way.

Golann D. 1996. *Mediating legal disputes: Effective strategies*. Boston: Little, Brown. Excellent book aimed at legal audience.

Lax DA and JK Sebenius. 1986. *The manager as negotiator: Bargaining for cooperation and competitive gain.* New York: Free Press. One of the best books on negotiation. Describes the tension that exists in most negotiations between what the authors label "value creating" and "value claiming" behavior and makes suggestions for managing that tension.

Marcus L. 1995. *Renegotiating health care: Resolving conflict to build collaboration.* San Francisco: Jossey-Bass.

Moore CW. 1996. *The mediation process: Practical strategies for resolving conflict.* 2nd ed. San Francisco: Jossey-Bass. Sets the standard for other works about mediation. Combines a clear description of the basics of the mediation process with discussion of more sophisticated issues.

Shell GR. 1999. *Bargaining for advantage: Negotiating strategies for reasonable people.* New York: Viking. About negotiations. Very readable and full of important insights.

Stulberg JB. 1987. *Taking charge/managing conflict.* Lexington, MA: Lexington Books. Excellent basic guide to conflict resolution and mediation.

Susskind LE, S McKearnan, and J Thomas-Larmer, eds. 1999. *The consensus building handbook: A comprehensive guide to reaching agreement.* Thousand Oaks, CA: Sage. Theory and case studies of complex, multiparty disputes.

Ury WL and JM Brett. 1991. *Getting past no.* New York: Bantam Books. Excellent discussion of what to do when the going gets tough.

Ury WL, JM Brett, and SB Goldberg. 1988. *Getting disputes resolved: Designing systems to cut the costs of conflict.* San Francisco: Jossey-Bass. Draws on the experiences of the authors and presents a method of analyzing the dispute resolution process and guidelines to implementing effective systems in business and other settings. Good analysis of the relationship between interests, rights, and power as a means for settling disputes.

## Loose-leaf

Cole SR, NH Rogers, and CA McEwen. 1994. 2nd ed. *Mediation: Law, policy, and practice.* Loose-leaf. St. Paul, Minn.: West Group. (Updated annually with replacement pages and cumulative supplement.) Comprehensive guide to mediation practice and legislation.

## Journals

*Alternatives.* Published monthly by CPR Institute for Dispute Resolution. Many of the best articles are available online at www.cpradr.org

*Conflict Resolution Quarterly.*

*Harvard Negotiation Law Review.*

*Journal of Dispute Resolution.* University of Missouri-Columbia School of Law.

*Mediation Quarterly.* Sponsored by the Association for Conflict Resolution.

*Negotiation Journal.* Published in cooperation with the Harvard Program on Negotiation, an Inter-University Consortium, Kluwer Academic/Plenum Publishers. Available online at www.kluweronline.com/issn/0748-4526/current

*Ohio State Journal on Dispute Resolution.*

## Web Sites

<www.ACResolution.org>
<www.crinfo.org> Maintained by Conflict Research Consortium, University of Colorado, and funded by the William and Flora Hewlett Foundation.

# *References*

Adams JL. 2001. *Conceptual blockbusting: A guide to better ideas.* 4th ed. Cambridge, MA: Perseus.

Allred KG. 2000. Anger and retaliation in conflict: The role of attribution. In *The handbook of conflict resolution: Theory and practice,* ed. M Deutsch and PT Coleman, 249–50. San Francisco: Jossey-Bass.

American Society for Bioethics and Humanities. 1998. *Core competencies for bioethics consultation.* Glenview, IL: American Society for Bioethics and Humanities.

Arrow K, RH Mnookin, L Ross, A Tversky, and R Wilson, eds. 1995. *Barriers to conflict resolution.* New York: W. W. Norton.

Beauchamp TL and JF Childress. 1994. *Principles of biomedical ethics.* 4th ed. New York: Oxford University Press.

Blustein J, LF Post, and N Dubler. 2002. *Ethics for health care organizations: Theory, case studies, and tools.* New York: United Hospital Fund.

Bush RAB. 1989. Efficiency and protection, or empowerment and recognition? The mediator's role and ethical standards in mediation. *Florida Law Review* 41:253.

Bush RAB and JP Folger. 1994. *The promise of mediation: Responding to conflict through empowerment and recognition.* San Francisco: Jossey-Bass.

Chew PK. 2001. *The conflict and culture reader.* New York: New York University Press.

Della Noce DJ. 2001. Mediation as a transformative process. In *Designing mediation: Approaches to training and practice within a transformative framework,* ed. JP Folger and RAB Bush, 71–84. New York: Institute for the Study of Conflict Transformation.

Dubler NN. 1995. The doctor-proxy relationship: The neglected connection. *Kennedy Institute of Ethics Journal* 5:289–306.

Dubler NN and LJ Marcus. 1994. *Mediating bioethical disputes.* New York: United Hospital Fund.

Fadiman A. 1998. *The spirit catches you and you fall down: A Hmong child, her American doctors, and the collision of two cultures.* New York: Farrar, Straus and Giroux.

Fisher R and W Ury. 1981. *Getting to yes: Negotiating agreement without giving in.* New York: Penguin.

Guthrie C. 2003. Panacea or Pandora's box? The costs of options in negotiation. *Iowa Law Review* 88:601.

Hickson GB, EW Clayton, PB Githens, and FA Sloan. 1992. Factors that prompted families to file medical malpractice claims following perinatal injuries. *Journal of the American Medical Association* 267:1359–63.

Hyman CS. 2002. Conversation with Carol Liebman, July.

Kimmel PR. 2000. Culture and conflict. In *The handbook of conflict resolution: Theory and practice*, ed. M Deutsch and PT Coleman, 453–74. San Francisco: Jossey-Bass.

Kressel K. 2000. Mediation. In *The handbook of conflict resolution: Theory and practice*, ed. M Deutsch and PT Coleman, 522–45. San Francisco: Jossey-Bass.

Lax DA and JK Sebenius. 1986. *The manager as negotiator: Bargaining for cooperation and competitive gain.* New York: Free Press.

Levine C and C Zuckerman. 1999. The trouble with families: Toward an ethic of accommodation. *Annals of Internal Medicine* 130(2):148–52.

Levinson W, DL Roter, JP Mullooly, VT Dull, and RM Frankel. 1997. Physician-patient communication: The relationship with malpractice claims among primary care physicians and surgeons. *Journal of the American Medical Association* 277:553–59.

Lewicki RJ and C Wiethoff. 2000. Trust, trust development, and trust repair. In *The handbook of conflict resolution: Theory and practice*, ed. M Deutsch and PT Coleman, 86–107. San Francisco: Jossey-Bass.

Love L and J Stulberg. 1996. Practice guidelines for co-mediation: Making certain that two heads are better than one. *Mediation Quarterly* 13(3):179–89.

Marcus L. 1992. Training session, Montefiore Medical Center, New York, Fall.

Menkel-Meadow C. 2001. Aha? Is creativity possible in legal problem solving and teachable in legal education? *Harvard Negotiation Law Review* 6:97.

Mnookin RH, SR Peppet, and AS Tulumello. 2000. *Beyond winning.* Cambridge, MA: Harvard University Press.

Moore CW. 1996. *The mediation process: Practical strategies for resolving conflict.* 2d ed. San Francisco: Jossey-Bass.

Pope SG. 1993. *Goals of questions.* On file with author.

Powell T. 1999. Extubating Mrs. K: Psychological aspects of surrogate decision making. *Journal of Law, Medicine & Ethics* 27(1):81–86.

Riskin LL. 1984. Toward new standards for the neutral lawyer in mediation. *Arizona Law Review* 26:329–62.

———. 1996. Understanding mediators' orientations, strategies, and techniques: A grid for the perplexed. *Harvard Negotiation Law Review* 1:7–49.

———. 2003. Who decides what? Rethinking the grid of mediator orientations. *Dispute Resolution Magazine* 9(22):22–25.

Ross JW, JW Glaser, D Rasinski-Gregory, JM Gibson, and C Bayley. 1993. *Health care ethics committees: The next generation.* San Francisco: Jossey-Bass.

Shaw M. 2000. Mediation training at Qinhua University, Beijing, June.

Shell GR. 1999. *Bargaining for advantage: Negotiating strategies for reasonable people.* New York: Viking.

Stone D, B Patton, and S Heen. 1999. *Difficult conversations: How to discuss what matters most.* New York: Viking.

Stulberg J. 1981. The theory and practice of mediation: A reply to Professor Susskind. *Vermont Law Review* 6:85.

Susskind LE. 1981. Environmental mediation and the accountability problem. *Vermont Law Review* 6:1.

Symposium: The doctor-proxy relationship. 1999. Symposium editor, N Dubler. *Journal of Law, Medicine & Ethics* 27(1):5–86.

Thompson L and J Nadler. 2000. Judgmental biases in conflict and how to overcome them. In *The handbook of conflict resolution: Theory and practice,* ed. M Deutsch and PT Coleman, 213–35. San Francisco: Jossey-Bass.

# About the Authors

**Nancy Neveloff Dubler** is the Director of the Division of Bioethics, Department of Epidemiology and Population Health, Montefiore Medical Center and Professor of Epidemiology and Population Health at the Albert Einstein College of Medicine. Ms. Dubler founded the Bioethics Consultation Service at Montefiore Medical Center in 1978, as a support for analysis of difficult cases presenting ethical issues in the health care setting. She is Director of the Certificate Program in Bioethics and Medical Humanities, conducted jointly by Montefiore Medical Center/Albert Einstein College of Medicine and The Hartford Institute of Geriatric Nursing at New York University. She lectures extensively and is the author of numerous articles and books on termination of care, home care and long-term care, geriatrics, prison and jail health care, ethics committees and consultation, and AIDS.

**Carol B. Liebman** is a Clinical Professor at Columbia Law School, where she is the Director of the Columbia Law School Mediation Clinic and the Negotiation Workshop. She also teaches professional ethics. She has mediated cases involving discrimination, medical malpractice, family issues, public agencies, community disputes, business conflicts, and educational institutions and is a nationally recognized speaker and trainer in conflict resolution. She has designed and presented mediation training for a variety of groups including the Certification Program in Bioethics of Montefiore Medical Center, Albert Einstein College of Medicine; New York's First Department, Appellate Division, Attorney Disciplinary Committee; and the Association of the Bar of the City of New York. She has taught about negotiation and mediation in Vietnam, Brazil, Israel, and China. Professor Liebman is currently working on a project funded by the Pew Charitable Trusts to explore ways mediation and conflict resolution techniques can be used in discussions of adverse medical events.

# Index

retrospective case consultation, 7
right to know, conflicting perspectives on, 150,
    151, 175–176, 179, 180
right to refuse care, xv, 106, 107
risk manager
    in absence of agreement, 75
    as bioethics mediator, 42
    and mediator, relations between, 198, 200
    position of, in role play, 161, 169
    role of, 14, 102, 199–200
Riskin, Leonard, 24
role plays
    at-risk pregnancy, 147–152, 173–185
    discharge planning for dying patient,
        139–145
    dying adolescent, 163–170
    giving feedback for, 136–138
    HIV and postsurgical complications,
        153–162, 187–215
    using, 135–136
role reversal, 95

scarce resources, issue of, 16–17, 117, 129
schizophrenia, 109
seating arrangements, in bioethics mediation
    meeting, 58
SICU. *See* Surgical Intensive Care Unit
silence, allowing, 94
social workers
    and anticipatory bereavement counsel-
        ing, 56
    and dying patient's family, support for, 103,
        104
    as participants in bioethics mediation, 48
    position of, in role play, 140–141, 142
    as potential bioethics mediators, 42
solutions, shaping, 73–74
speakers, order of, decision regarding,
    190–191
stenosis, 109
stroking, 93, 138, 194
suffering. *See* pain and suffering
suicide. *See* physician-assisted suicide
summarizing, 87–89, 179, 202–203, 209, 213
    of medical facts, 87, 192, 193–194
    of options, 182–183

Supreme Court, on physician-assisted sui-
    cide, 49
surgeons, time and cost constraints on, 112
Surgical Intensive Care Unit (SICU), 117,
    121–122
Swartz, Barbara, 105n, 112n

termination of care. *See also* do not resuscitate
    (DNR) order
    ambivalence about, 103–104
    vs. assisted suicide, 48
    delaying decision about, 105–106
    hospital policies regarding, 197
    New York State law on, 159, 161, 200–201
    patient's right to, xv, 106, 107
    reasons for, 55
    supporting patient's decision regarding, 105
therapeutic counseling, vs. bioethics media-
    tion, 46
time constraints
    assessing, 53
    in bioethics mediation, 27
    on clinical care coordinators, 112
    on surgeons, 112
training, mediation, xv, 85
transparency, of bioethics mediator, 131, 132,
    176
trust, building, 60

uncertainty, medical, 63
United Hospital Fund, xv
Ury, W., 38

ventilator. *See* intubation
visiting hours and rules
    compromise about, 123–124
    conflict over, 119
    in Surgical Intensive Care Unit, 122
voice, of mediator, 199, 209
Von Recklinghausen's disease, 47

working hypothesis
    developing, 70–72
    examples of, 152, 162, 170, 198
    revising, 72, 213
    testing, 71